AF790724

Magnetic Nanomaterials

Innovation for cancer theranostics

Online at: https://doi.org/10.1088/978-0-7503-6335-8

IPEM–IOP Series in Physics and Engineering in Medicine and Biology

Editorial Advisory Board Members

Frank Verhaegen
Maastro Clinic, The Netherlands

Carmel Caruana
University of Malta, Malta

Penelope Allisy-Roberts
formerly of BIPM, Sèvres, France

Rory Cooper
University of Pittsburgh, PA, USA

Alicia El Haj
University of Birmingham, UK

Kwan Hoong Ng
University of Malaya, Malaysia

John Hossack
University of Virginia, USA

Tingting Zhu
University of Oxford, UK

Dennis Schaart
TU Delft, The Netherlands

Indra J Das
Northwestern University Feinberg School of Medicine, USA

About the Series

The series in Physics and Engineering in Medicine and Biology will allow the Institute of Physics and Engineering in Medicine (IPEM) to enhance its mission to 'advance physics and engineering applied to medicine and biology for the public good'.

It is focused on key areas including, but not limited to:

- clinical engineering
- diagnostic radiology
- informatics and computing
- magnetic resonance imaging
- nuclear medicine
- physiological measurement
- radiation protection
- radiotherapy
- rehabilitation engineering
- ultrasound and non-ionising radiation.

A number of IPEM–IOP titles are being published as part of the EUTEMPE Network Series for Medical Physics Experts.

A full list of titles published in this series can be found here: https://iopscience.iop.org/bookListInfo/physics-engineering-medicine-biology-series.

Magnetic Nanomaterials

Innovation for cancer theranostics

Sudip Mukherjee
School of Biomedical Engineering, Indian Institute of Technology (BHU), Varanasi, Uttar Pradesh, India

Vijay Sagar Madamsetty
Lifeedit Therapeutics, Durham, NC, 27701, United States of America

Lipi Pradhan
School of Biomedical Engineering, Indian Institute of Technology (BHU), Varanasi, Uttar Pradesh, India

Anjali Upadhyay
School of Biomedical Engineering, Indian Institute of Technology (BHU), Varanasi, Uttar Pradesh, India

Devyani Yenurkar
School of Biomedical Engineering, Indian Institute of Technology (BHU), Varanasi, Uttar Pradesh, India

IOP Publishing, Bristol, UK

© IOP Publishing Ltd 2025. All rights, including for text and data mining (TDM), artificial intelligence (AI) training, and similar technologies, are reserved.

This book is available under the terms of the IOP-Standard Books License

No part of this publication may be reproduced, stored in a retrieval system, subjected to any form of TDM or used for the training of any AI systems or similar technologies, or transmitted in any form or by any means, electronic, mechanical, photocopying, recording or otherwise, without the prior permission of the publisher, or as expressly permitted by law or under terms agreed with the appropriate rights organization. Certain types of copying may be permitted in accordance with the terms of licences issued by the Copyright Licensing Agency, the Copyright Clearance Centre and other reproduction rights organizations.

Permission to make use of IOP Publishing content other than as set out above may be sought at permissions@ioppublishing.org.

Sudip Mukherjee, Vijay Sagar Madamsetty, Lipi Pradhan, Anjali Upadhyay and Devyani Yenurkar have asserted their right to be identified as the authors of this work in accordance with sections 77 and 78 of the Copyright, Designs and Patents Act 1988.

ISBN 978-0-7503-6335-8 (ebook)
ISBN 978-0-7503-6333-4 (print)
ISBN 978-0-7503-6336-5 (myPrint)
ISBN 978-0-7503-6334-1 (mobi)

DOI 10.1088/978-0-7503-6335-8

Version: 20250501

IOP ebooks

British Library Cataloguing-in-Publication Data: A catalogue record for this book is available from the British Library.

Published by IOP Publishing, wholly owned by The Institute of Physics, London

IOP Publishing, No.2 The Distillery, Glassfields, Avon Street, Bristol, BS2 0GR, UK

US Office: IOP Publishing, Inc., 190 North Independence Mall West, Suite 601, Philadelphia, PA 19106, USA

Contents

Preface

Magnetic nanoparticles (MNPs) have emerged as a dynamic and rapidly evolving field within nanomedicine that has revolutionized cancer theranostics. This book focuses on the recent advancements in MNP research, highlighting their methods of synthesis and their biomedical application including their role in targeted drug delivery, magnetic hyperthermia therapy, diagnosis, and imaging for cancer.

Acknowledgments

We want to acknowledge the director of the Indian Institute of Technology (BHU), Varanasi, India, for continuous support.

Author biographies

Sudip Mukherjee

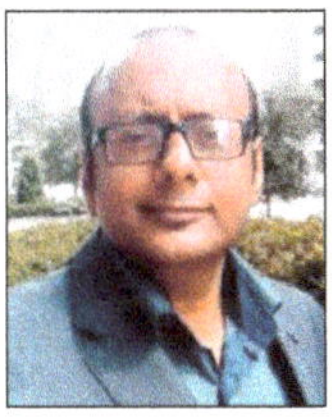

Sudip Mukherjee, PhD, MRSC, is an Assistant Professor of School of Biomedical Engineering at the Indian Institute of Technology, BHU (IIT BHU). Dr Mukherjee completed his PhD from CSIR-IICT, Hyderabad in 2017, following which he worked at Rice University, Houston till 2022 as a postdoctoral research associate. His research interests include the development of advanced biomaterials for cell therapy and drug/gene delivery in various rare genetic disorders (Type-1 diabetes, Gaucher's disease, amyotrophic lateral sclerosis (ALS), Duchene muscular dystrophy, etc), fibrosis, tissue regeneration, cancer theranostics, and other inflammatory diseases. He has published over 80 research (*Nature Biomedical Engineering, Advanced Materials, Science Advances, Theranostics, Chemical Science* etc) and review articles and has 24 US/INDIAN patents filed/granted with total citations over 6700 with 'h' index of '41' and 'i' index of '62'. Dr Mukherjee has published six books with reputed publishers (Springer, IOP, Elsevier etc). Multiple technologies (LOCOcyte) are licensed and have been part of cell engineering-based therapies that are currently under clinical trials (Phase I/II) for advanced peritoneal cancers. Dr Mukherjee received several awards including Houston Methodist-Rice University travel grant, Sakura Exchange Visiting grant, KVRAO young scientist award, multiple best poster awards etc. Dr Mukherjee serves as an Associate Editor for *BMC Cancer* and *Frontiers in Chemistry* and is a member of Royal Society of Chemistry (RSC), UK; American Chemical Society (ACS), USA and Society for Biomaterials and Artificial Organs, India. From 2020–2024, Dr Mukherjee was included in the prestigious list of World's Top 2% scientists jointly published by the Stanford University and Elsevier five consecutive times.

Dr Vijay Sagar Madamsetty

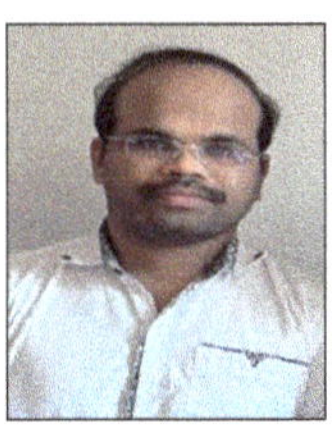

Dr Vijay Sagar Madamsetty earned his PhD from the CSIR–Indian Institute of Chemical Technology and is currently a Senior Scientist in the U.S. biopharmaceutical industry. He previously spent six years at the Mayo Clinic College of Medicine and two years at CSL Seqirus, where his research focused on developing lipid nanoparticles for the targeted delivery of therapeutics, gene editing tools, and vaccines. In his current role, he leads efforts in the formulation and optimization of lipid nanoparticle-based drug delivery systems, supporting both preclinical and clinical development programs. Dr Madamsetty has authored 29 peer-reviewed publications and remains deeply committed to advancing the fields of nanomedicine, drug delivery, and pharmaceutical innovation.

Lipi Pradhan

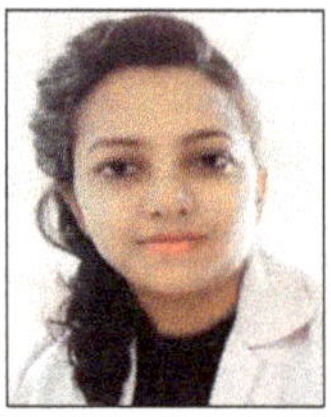

Lipi Pradhan is a research scholar currently pursuing her PhD degree at the School of Biomedical Engineering, IIT BHU She earned her MSc in Zoology at the Department of Zoology, Ranchi University. Her research interests include designing cell-based therapies for treating rare genetic disorders and the green synthesis of nanoparticles for various biomedical applications.

Anjali Upadhyay

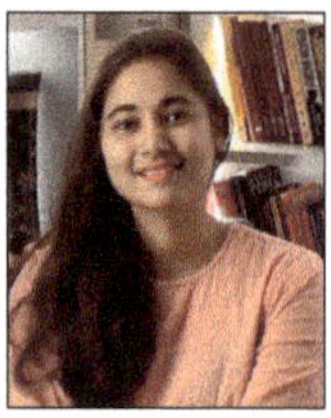

Anjali Upadhyay is a research scholar currently pursuing her PhD at the School of Biomedical Engineering, IIT BHU. She completed her master's degree (MSc) at the University of Allahabad (Department of Zoology). Her research interests include inorganic biomaterials for antifibrotic, antibacterial, and antibiofilm applications.

Devyani Yenurkar

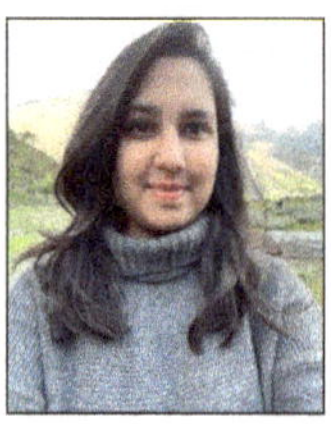

Devyani Yenurkar is a Prime Minister's Research Fellow (PMRF) in the School of Biomedical Engineering, IIT BHU. She received her master's degree in pharmacy (pharmaceutics) from SNDT University, Mumbai. Her current research interests include working with nanomaterials for their potential applications in the field of blood anticoagulation and thrombosis.

Chapter 1

Introduction to magnetic nanomaterials

Magnetic nanomaterials (MNs) have emerged as a pivotal innovation in nanotechnology, gaining substantial attention due to their effective application in the biomedical field. These remarkable materials possess unique characteristics, including a uniform particle size that maximizes surface area and enhances interaction with biological systems. Their inducible magnetic moments enable precise control over their movement and positioning within the body, making targeted therapy possible. Furthermore, their superior adsorption kinetics enhance their ability to bind with therapeutic agents efficiently. In this chapter, various types of magnetic nanoparticles (MNPs), their properties, and their applications in different biological fields are discussed.

In recent years, a growing body of research has illuminated the profound potential of nanotechnology in biomedicine, particularly in diagnosing and treating various human diseases. The unique properties of MNPs and their advancements in the field warrant their utilization in various biomedical applications. This convergence opens up a wealth of exhilarating opportunities for researchers to explore and develop innovative nanomaterials [1–4]. Through a variety of cutting-edge processes, scientists are uncovering novel materials that hold great promise for applications across medicine, environmental science, and beyond, pushing the boundaries of what is possible in both nanotechnology and biological research [5–7]. MNPs have emerged as a pivotal innovation in the realm of nanotechnology, gaining substantial attention due to their effective application in the treatment of lymphatic nodes and the management of metastasized tumors [8–12]. These remarkable materials possess a range of unique characteristics, including a uniform particle size that maximizes surface area, allowing for enhanced interaction with biological systems [13–16]. Their inducible magnetic moments enable precise control over their movement and positioning within the body, making targeted therapy possible [17–20]. Additionally, MNPs are designed to be nontoxic and biocompatible, ensuring safety when used in medical applications [21–24]. Furthermore, their

doi:10.1088/978-0-7503-6335-8ch1 © IOP Publishing Ltd 2025. All rights, including for text and data mining (TDM), artificial intelligence (AI) training, and similar technologies, are reserved.

superior adsorption kinetics enhance their ability to bind with therapeutic agents efficiently [15, 24–26]. Collectively, these properties are driving rapid advancements in the development of MNPs for specific and compelling biomedical uses [27–29]. MNPs are unique nanomaterials characterized by their metallic cores, usually composed of materials such as iron oxide, cobalt, or nickel [30–33]. These cores are stabilized and functionalized by an outer shell often enhanced with various functional groups, such as polymers, biological molecules, or silica, to improve their biocompatibility and target specificity [8, 15, 34–38].

Typically, MNPs are less than 100 nanometers in size, which allows them to interact effectively with biological systems at the cellular and molecular levels [18, 39–42]. They can be synthesized from a wide range of magnetically active materials, enabling customization based on specific application requirements [43–46]. MNPs have gained significant attention in the medical field due to their versatile applications [43, 47–49]. They are particularly valuable in targeted drug delivery, enhancing the precision of drug delivery to specific cells and improving MRI contrast for better diagnostics [31, 50–53]. Additionally, MNPs are used in cancer therapy and biosensing, making them a transformative tool in modern medicine with the potential to enhance patient outcomes [8, 54–56]. In the context of cancer treatment, MNPs play a vital role by enabling targeted drug delivery systems. By attaching therapeutic agents to the surface of MNPs, clinicians can concentrate treatment at tumor sites while minimizing side effects on healthy tissues [57]. This targeted approach protects the patient's overall health and enhances the efficacy of the treatment [58, 59]. Figure 1.1 describes the applications of these MNPs in cancer therapy.

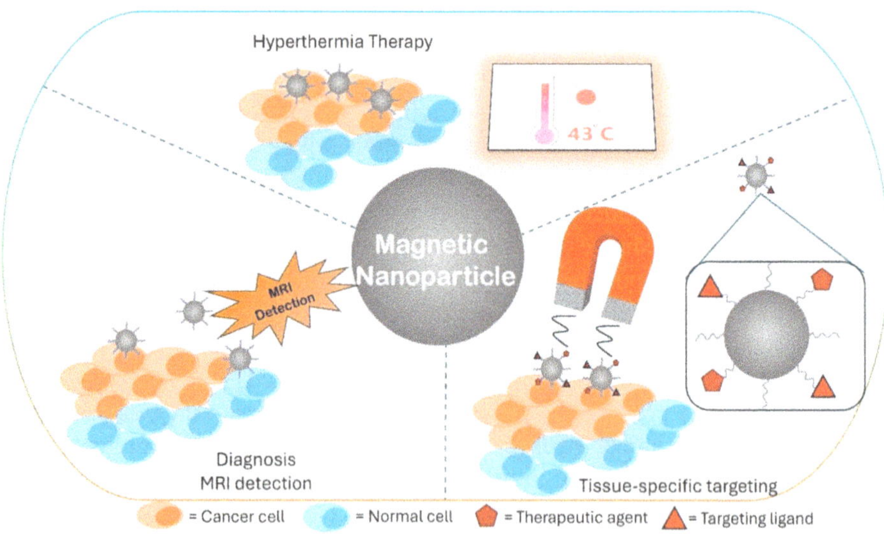

Figure 1.1. Examples of MNP use in cancer detection and treatment. Drug delivery, diagnosis, and hyperthermic therapy. Adapted with permission from [83]. CC BY-NC-ND 3.0.

1. **Hyperthermia:** MNP technology has the ability to produce localized heat when subjected to alternating magnetic fields [56, 60]. This characteristic is particularly valuable in the field of cancer treatment, as it enables the targeted destruction of cancer cells without significantly harming the surrounding healthy tissue [61, 62]. By precisely controlling the magnetic field, healthcare professionals can focus the heat generated by the MNPs directly on tumor sites, effectively raising the temperature in those localized areas [14, 63, 64]. This targeted hyperthermic treatment increases the chances of eradicating cancerous cells while preserving the integrity and function of adjacent healthy cells, thereby reducing potential side effects associated with conventional treatments [65–67].
2. **Drug delivery agents:** MNPs represent an advanced approach to drug delivery, offering a method for precise and targeted treatment [68–71]. These tiny carriers can be functionalized by attaching therapeutic agents directly to their surfaces, allowing them to seek out and bind specifically to cancerous cells [10, 13, 72, 73]. This targeted delivery system not only enhances the effectiveness of the treatment by ensuring that the drugs are concentrated where they are needed most, but also significantly reduces potential side effects that often accompany conventional chemotherapy. By minimizing damage to healthy tissues, MNPs pave the way for more effective and safe cancer therapies [44].
3. **Imaging:** MNPs serve as effective contrast agents in a variety of imaging techniques, particularly in magnetic resonance imaging (MRI) [44, 74]. Due to their unique magnetic properties, these nanoparticles significantly improve the visibility of different tissues and abnormalities within the body [69, 74, 75]. By enhancing the contrast in MRI scans, MNPs facilitate more accurate identification and diagnosis of conditions at an early stage [76]. This capability is instrumental in guiding treatment decisions and improving patient outcomes, as it allows for timely intervention and monitoring of various diseases [76]. Additionally, researchers are continuously exploring new formulations of MNPs to further enhance their imaging efficacy and safety in clinical applications [77].
4. **Detection:** MNPs are increasingly utilized in biosensors for the sensitive detection of biomolecules, including proteins and nucleic acids [77, 78]. This capability is crucial for various disease diagnosis and monitoring applications [78]. By employing MNPs, biosensors can achieve enhanced sensitivity and specificity, allowing for the rapid identification of biomarkers associated with specific diseases [54, 79]. This technology plays a vital role in early diagnosis, treatment planning, and ongoing health monitoring, ultimately improving patient outcomes and facilitating effective healthcare interventions [80].
5. **Extraction of biomolecules:** MNPs have distinct magnetic characteristics that facilitate the effective isolation and purification of biomolecules; these characteristics are crucial for various applications in research settings and clinical laboratories [48, 49, 81]. Due to their surface modifications, these

nanoparticles can efficiently bind to specific biomolecules, allowing for targeted separation from complex biological mixtures [81, 82].

Furthermore, the versatility of MNPs allows them to be used in a wide range of biomedical applications, including imaging, diagnostics, and the development of biosensors [84]. Their ability to be customized for specific tasks makes them valuable in advancing personalized medicine, where treatments can be tailored to individual patients based on their unique biological profiles [16, 85]. Through ongoing research and innovation, MNPs continue to significantly contribute to the evolution of cancer therapies and the broader field of biomedical science.

Due to their unique properties, MNPs are increasingly important in various analytical applications [86, 87]. They serve as effective magnetic carriers in separation processes, facilitating the isolation and purification of specific biomolecules [88]. Additionally, MNPs are employed as biosensors, which enhance the detection of molecular recognition events, allowing the identification of specific proteins or pathogens at very low concentrations [89, 90]. In medical imaging, these nanoparticles act as contrast agents in MRI, improving the clarity and detail of the images obtained, which is essential for accurate diagnosis [91].

Their role in cancer treatment is particularly significant and multifaceted [92]. One of their main therapeutic applications involves the targeted delivery of drugs and bioactive compounds directly into cancer cells [93]. This targeted approach minimizes damage to healthy tissues and maximizes the therapeutic effects on tumors [47]. Furthermore, MNPs are utilized in hyperthermic treatments, where they are directed to tumor sites and heated using an external magnetic field [94, 95]. This localized heating can help to destroy cancer cells and enhance the effectiveness of concurrent therapies [60, 96, 97]. The diverse capabilities and innovative applications of MNPs are paving the way for groundbreaking advancements in cancer diagnostics and treatment. These tiny, multifunctional particles hold great promise, as they enhance the accuracy of detecting tumors and enable targeted therapies that effectively combat cancer while minimizing damage to healthy tissues. As research continues to evolve, MNPs are expected to play a crucial role in transforming the oncology landscape [8].

In recent years, the field of MNPs has made significant strides in transitioning from theoretical research settings to practical clinical applications. This progress has sparked considerable interest among scientists and researchers eager to explore the potential benefits and uses of MNPs in medicine and biotechnology [30]. Iron oxide nanoparticles (IONPs) have garnered particular attention among the various types of nanoparticles being studied [98, 99]. Researchers have extensively examined these nanoparticles due to their unique magnetic properties and biocompatibility [100]. One of their defining characteristics is that they do not retain any magnetization once the external magnetic field is removed. This property is highly advantageous for various applications, as it allows for precise control over the particles without the risk of unwanted magnetic interactions once treatment is complete [101, 102].

IONPs are being explored for a wide range of biomedical applications [100, 103]. For example, they are utilized in targeted drug delivery systems, where they can be magnetically guided to specific sites within the body, enhancing the effectiveness of treatments while minimizing side effects [104]. Additionally, their imaging capabilities make them valuable in MRI, improving the contrast of images and aiding in diagnosing various conditions [105]. Furthermore, these nanoparticles hold promise in cancer therapy, where they can be used in hyperthermic treatment, in which localized heating facilitated by an alternating magnetic field helps to target and destroy cancerous cells. The growing body of research into IONPs highlights their potential to revolutionize medical treatments and diagnostics, presenting a promising frontier in nanomedicine. For most MNPs, the metallic core comprises iron- or iron-oxide-based compounds [18, 106].

The presence of the magnetic core primarily enables these MNPs to be manipulated using magnetic field gradients. IONPs (Fe_3O_4 and Fe_2O_3) have been widely applied for *in vitro* diagnosis and, more recently, for other applications, due to their easy functionalization with polymers and other materials [107]. Further, the US Food and Drug Administration (US FDA) approved iron oxide MNPs (ferumoxytol, also known as Feraheme®) for treating adult iron deficiency anemia [108]. Additionally, iron oxide MNPs are also used by clinicians as off-label MRI contrast agents [109]. Moreover, the European Medicines Agency (EMA) has also approved the use of iron oxide MNPs as MRI contrast agents. Ferucarbotran, also known as Resovist®, is one example of an EMA-approved contrast agent [110]. Other MNPs are also approved for GBM and interstitial prostate cancer in Europe and the US [111, 112]. These clinical advancements of MNPs have paved the way for the current biomedical research field's attention to their unique magnetic properties. In the following sections, we will briefly explore the historical background of MNPs, overview the diverse categories of MNPs, and highlight the innovative cancer therapies that leverage these unique materials. In addition, we will discuss the challenges of developing and applying MNPs in medical settings, paving the way for deeper discussions in future sections. Our goal is to examine the complexities of working with MNPs while thoroughly examining the cutting-edge advancements in this field.

1.1 History of metallic nanoparticles

Nanoparticle-based structures were ingeniously employed by the Romans in the fourth century AD, highlighting an extraordinary instance of ancient nanotechnology [113]. These innovative techniques led to the creation of stunning 'luster' ceramic glazes, which shimmered and sparkled due to the incorporation of silver (Ag) or copper (Cu) nanoparticles [114]. These captivating glazes were popular in the Islamic world and gained prominence throughout Europe [115]. By the 16th century, skilled Italian artisans harnessed the power of metal nanoparticles to craft exquisite Renaissance pottery, resulting in richly adorned pieces that reflected artistry and scientific mastery [116]. One of the most fascinating and ancient examples of nanotechnology is the remarkable Lycurgus Cup, which resides in the esteemed collection of the British Museum. This exquisite piece of glasswork is renowned as an early form of dichroic glass, which brilliantly shifts its color depending on the surrounding lighting conditions [113]. Intrigued by this optical phenomenon, scientists employed transmission electron microscopy (TEM) to examine the cup's unique properties and unravel the mystery behind its captivating dichroism. The striking interplay of colors, displaying hues that seem to change when viewed from different angles, arises from nanoparticles embedded within the glass matrix, with diameters ranging between 50 and 100 nanometers [117, 118]. Further analysis using x-ray techniques revealed that these intriguing nanoparticles comprise a carefully crafted alloy of silver and gold (Ag–Au), with a specific ratio of approximately 7:3, alongside about 10% copper (Cu). The stunning red color exhibited by the gold nanoparticles results from their ability to absorb light at around 520 nanometers. These larger particles interact with light to generate a vivid red-purple hue [113].

In contrast, the playful green color emitted by the cup results from light scattering by colloidal dispersions of silver nanoparticles, which exceed 40 nanometers in size, creating a brilliant visual effect that enchants viewers [113]. The Lycurgus Cup is a testament to ancient artistry and a remarkable illustration of nanotechnological principles [119]. This phenomenon parallels the characteristics observed in late medieval church windows, where the integration of gold (Au) and silver (Ag) nanoparticles into the glass matrix results in strikingly vibrant red and yellow hues [113]. These colors arise from the unique optical properties of the nanoparticles, which can scatter and absorb light in specific ways, enhancing the overall aesthetic of the glass [113, 120]. In the 19th century, the concept of colloidal gold was notably advanced by Michael Faraday, who made his discovery in the 1850s. His work laid the foundation for understanding how metal nanoparticles could be suspended in a liquid medium, influencing science and art [121, 122]. Following this, in 1908, physicist Gustav Mie provided a groundbreaking theoretical framework that demonstrated how light interacts with metal nanoparticles. His research marked a significant development in the field, ultimately paving the way for the exploration of metal-based nanotechnology and its numerous applications in various industries, including imaging, sensing, and therapeutics [123].

In 1986, physicists Gerd Binnig and Heinrich Rohrer received the prestigious Nobel Prize for their groundbreaking invention of the scanning tunneling microscope (STM) [124]. This remarkable instrument transformed the landscape of nanotechnology, allowing scientists to visualize surfaces at the atomic level with unprecedented clarity. The STM set a new standard for imaging and manipulating matter on a nanoscale and laid the foundation for subsequent innovations, such as the atomic force microscope (AFM) and the scanning probe microscope (SPM) [124–126]. Today, these advanced tools are indispensable for researchers, enabling detailed exploration and understanding of materials and biological systems at the nanoscale [127]. Spanning several decades, extensive investigations into the applications of nanotechnology within the biological sciences have revealed its remarkable capabilities in areas such as disease diagnosis, targeted drug delivery, and advanced molecular imaging, all of which have produced promising outcomes. One of the most exciting developments in this field is in nano-oncology, where groundbreaking strides have been made to enhance the efficacy of conventional chemotherapy drugs for a diverse array of aggressive cancers [128]. Nano-oncology uniquely leverages the principles of nanoscience, utilizing tiny, engineered particles to navigate the complexities of cancer treatment more effectively [129]. Researchers are able to precisely target tumors using innovative nanosized carriers, which are tiny delivery systems designed to transport therapeutic agents directly to cancerous cells [130]. This advanced approach enhances the accuracy of treatment and leads to significantly improved response rates, allowing for more effective and tailored interventions in cancer therapy [130].

Furthermore, this innovative approach offers the potential to markedly diminish the systemic toxicity often associated with traditional chemotherapy treatments. By focusing the delivery of medication directly to cancerous cells, this technique minimizes collateral damage to healthy tissues, representing a transformative leap in cancer therapy. The capacity to enhance treatment effectiveness while safeguarding the well-being of patients marks a significant advancement in the ongoing battle against cancer [131].

Types of MNPs: MNPs are categorized into several distinct types, each characterized by specific properties that set them apart. These types may include IONPs, noble metal nanoparticles, and various composite materials. Each category exhibits unique magnetic behaviors, size ranges, and surface characteristics, influencing their functionality and suitability for different applications [30, 132].

Understanding these classifications is crucial, as it allows researchers and practitioners to select the appropriate type of MNP for specific purposes, such as targeted drug delivery, MRI, environmental remediation, or data storage [76]. By grasping each type's distinct features and potential applications, we can optimize the use of MNPs in diverse fields, leading to advancements in technology and medicine [133].

Iron oxides, such as ferrite or IONPs (a type of MNP), possess a crystal structure characterized as either maghemite or magnetite [134]. These fascinating nanoparticles are extensively researched due to their unique properties and potential applications. When their size is reduced to below 128 nanometers, they enter a superparamagnetic state, allowing them to exhibit remarkable magnetic behavior when exposed to an external magnetic field [115, 135]. The enhancement of magnetic mobility in these ferrite nanoparticles can be achieved by carefully controlling the aggregation of individual nanoparticle clusters or magnetic nanobeads, improving performance in various applications [136]. Interestingly, once the external magnetic field is removed, these ferrite MNPs transform, reverting to a nonmagnetic state [137]. This ability to switch between magnetic and nonmagnetic states makes them particularly valuable in biomedical engineering, environmental remediation, and data storage technologies [104, 138].

Ferrites with a shell: ferrite MNPs are characterized by a relatively inert surface, which poses significant challenges when functionalizing them for specific applications [43]. This inertness limits their interaction with other substances, making it difficult to tailor their properties for use in various fields such as biomedicine, electronics, and materials science [139]. To address this limitation, one effective approach is to coat the surface of these nanoparticles with a layer of silica. This silica coating acts as a protective shell that enhances the stability of the ferrite nanoparticles and provides active sites for further functionalization [140]. Adding the silica layer can improve the nanoparticles' biocompatibility, facilitate their dispersion in solvents, and enable the attachment of biomolecules or other functional groups [140]. Due to this modification, the nanoparticles are called ferrites with a shell [141]. This designation highlights their dual composition: a magnetic core made of ferrite and a silica shell that expands their potential applications by allowing for further chemical modifications [141]. Such advancements can lead to more effective use in targeted drug delivery systems, MRI, and as catalysts in chemical reactions, among other applications [142].

The silica shell is highly versatile and can be readily modified to incorporate a variety of surface functional groups [143]. This modification is achieved through a covalent bond between organosilane compounds and the silica shell, allowing for tailored interactions and enhanced functionality in diverse applications [143]. Silica-shell-coated ferrite nanoparticles represent a remarkable advancement in nanotechnology, particularly when compared to conventional MNPs [144, 145]. One of their standout features is their impressive chemical stability, which ensures consistent performance in diverse environments alongside a narrow size distribution crucial for biomedical applications. This uniformity is vital, allowing for precise interactions in biological systems [144, 146]. These nanoparticles retain their superparamagnetic properties, which means they can be easily manipulated using external magnetic fields without clumping together, a phenomenon known as agglomeration. Their ability to remain colloidally stable makes them highly desirable for various applications where uniform dispersion is necessary [147]. The magnetic behavior of these nanoparticles is also tunable; by adjusting the cluster size, researchers can fine-tune their magnetic properties to meet specific requirements [148]. Besides these impressive qualities, the silica shell surrounding the nanoparticles is a versatile functionalization platform. This capability allows different chemical groups or biomolecules to be attached, significantly broadening their use in targeted drug delivery, imaging, and other innovative applications in biomedicine and materials science [149].

Metallic nanoparticles: metallic nanoparticles are tiny metal particles that range in size from 1 to 100 nm. They are used in various biomedical applications, including cancer theranostics [150, 151]. These nanoparticles have a large surface area relative to their size, a uniform and narrow size distribution, and improved bioavailability, making them advantageous for medical use. Many scientists have explored the potential of metallic nanoparticles in addressing various diseases, such as malaria and cancer diagnosis and treatment [152].

In addition to their biomedical applications, metallic nanoparticles have benefits in specific technical fields due to their higher magnetic moments [151]. However, they also have some drawbacks. For instance, they can be pyrophoric and reactive with oxidizing agents, which makes them challenging to handle and can lead to unwanted side reactions. Additionally, the formation of colloids containing metallic nanoparticles presents its own set of challenges [153].

Metallic with a shell: metallic shell nanoparticles, commonly called metallic nanoshells, consist of a nonconductive core encased in a metallic coating [154].

Recently, these nanoshells have gained considerable attention due to their remarkable optical properties. The metallic cores of these MNPs can be effectively protected through gentle oxidation and the use of surfactants, polymers, and precious metals [154, 155].

Cobalt (Co) nanoparticles develop an antiferromagnetic cobalt oxide (CoO) layer on their surface in an oxygen-rich environment [156]. The core radius and shell thickness can be easily adjusted for optimal tunability. These nanoparticles have various applications, including water desalination, purification, fluorescence enhancement in diagnostics, and biosensing [157].

Recent research has explored the impact of production methods and exchange bias in nanoparticles with a cobalt core, a cobalt oxide shell, and a gold outer shell. Significant advancements have also been made in synthesizing metals like iron and cobalt with a nonreactive graphene shell. These nanoparticles offer substantial advantages, such as enhanced magnetic properties and increased stability when exposed to acids, bases, and organic solvents [158]. Various types of metallic nanoshells, including gold (Au), iron (Fe), silver (Ag), and copper (Cu), have been extensively developed for biological imaging and therapeutic applications [106]. These nanoshells can be further modified with functional groups, such as targeting ligands, antibodies, anticancer drugs, genes, and imaging agents [106]. Several other combinations of MNPs have been developed to diagnose and treat cancer. As shown in figure 1.2, we will discuss magnetoliposomes, magnetomicelles, and magneto-polymeric carriers such as hydrogels or polymeric MNPs [159]. These MNPs are crucial for managing simultaneous thermochemotherapy, which is commonly administered intratumorally or intravenously.

Many researchers have demonstrated the efficacy of MNPs and drug-loaded nanoformulations in cancer diagnosis and therapy. The incorporation of MNPs further offers the possibility of guiding drugs by a magnetic field to target the tumor site in the body.

Magnetoliposomes: Magnetoliposomes are developed by incorporating MNPs into the liposome, either in the lipid membrane of the liposome's hydrophobic site or in the core of the liposome's hydrophilic site [160]. These liposomes are further loaded with anticancer drugs or imaging agents [160]. Additionally, temperature-sensitive magnetoliposomes can be developed using a specific lipid to achieve temperature-sensitive drug release controlled by an external magnetic field [161]. For example, researchers have engineered anticancer drug-loaded nanoliposomes as a novel approach to improve cancer therapy by harnessing the power of an external magnetic field [162]. These specialized delivery systems, magnetoliposomes, are designed to encapsulate the chemotherapeutic drug used to treat cancer. The application of an external magnetic field allows for targeted delivery of these magnetoliposomes to tumor sites, enhancing the accumulation of the drug where it is needed most [162, 163]. These magnetoliposomes have demonstrated promising results in cancer thermochemotherapy. This method combines thermal treatment with chemotherapy to increase the drug's effectiveness and reduce side effects on healthy tissues [164]. Additionally, their formulation exhibits excellent biocompatibility, which is crucial for minimizing adverse reactions when administered to

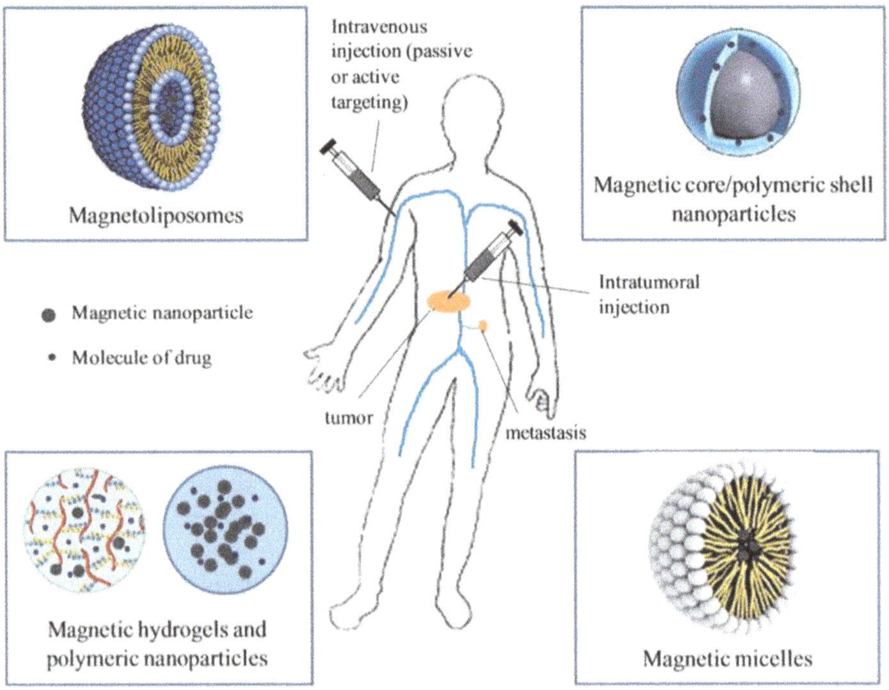

Figure 1.2. Types of MNPs used for cancer therapy. Adapted from [159]. CC BY 3.0.

patients [163]. Overall, this innovative approach has the potential to improve treatment outcomes in cancer therapy.

Recently, Ana *et al* developed an innovative treatment approach for colorectal cancer utilizing LGR5-functionalized biomimetic magnetoliposomes [165]. These advanced magnetoliposomes are specifically designed to carry two chemotherapeutic agents: oxaliplatin and fluorouracil (F-fluorouracil), which are well-known for their efficacy in treating colorectal cancer [165]. A key feature of this treatment is the leucine-rich repeat-containing G-protein coupled receptor 5 (LGR5), a membrane receptor that plays a crucial role in tissue-specific targeting. LGR5 is preferentially expressed on the surface of colorectal cancer cells, allowing for precise delivery of the therapeutic agents directly to the tumor site. This targeted approach enhances the treatment's effectiveness and minimizes potential side effects on healthy tissues. By leveraging the characteristics of LGR5, this cutting-edge therapy aims to improve patient outcomes in colorectal cancer treatment [165].

Magnetic micelles: Micelles comprise a hydrophilic head group and a hydrophobic tail, which spontaneously assemble in an aqueous solution [166]. This spontaneous assembly forms an aggregate with polar head groups facing the surrounding water and hydrophobic tails excluding water from the core [166]. These micelles help encapsulate hydrophobic drugs or MNPs in the micelle core [166]. Furthermore, these micelles extend the circulation time and enhance uptake via the enhanced permeability and retention (EPR) effect [166]. For instance, Song *et al* conducted a study in which they developed ferrimagnetic fluorescent micelles designed explicitly for image-guided magnetic hyperthermic therapy [167]. Their approach involved using a poly(D, L-lactide) (PLA)-based amphiphilic block copolymer, known for its biocompatibility and ability to form micelles. This copolymer effectively encapsulated highly ferrimagnetic MNPs, which provided therapeutic properties, along with ZnS/InP quantum dots used for imaging purposes. The team utilized a straightforward self-assembly method to create these micelles, yielding a stable and effective delivery system that integrated imaging and therapeutic capabilities. This innovative approach offers potential advancements in targeted cancer therapies by enhancing the precision of treatment delivery while monitoring the treatment's effectiveness in real time [167].

In a comparable investigation, Zhang *et al* focused on the development of manganese (Mn) coordination micelles that were explicitly engineered to encapsulate Chlorin-e6 (Ce6), Cas9 protein, and single guide RNA (sgRNA) [168]. This innovative approach aims to enhance the effectiveness of combination anticancer therapy. Incorporating Ce6, a photosensitizing agent, alongside genetic components like Cas9 and sgRNA, is intended to improve targeted gene editing and photodynamic therapy, ultimately leading to more effective treatment outcomes in cancer management. This multifaceted strategy represents a significant advancement in the field of cancer therapeutics [168]. In a separate research study, scientists engineered innovative magnetic micelles for gene therapy in breast cancer treatment. These micelles consist of a complex structure that includes polyethylene glycol (PEG), polyethylenimine (PEI), polylactic acid (PLA), and iron oxide (Fe_3O_4) nanoparticles combined with polycaprolactone (PCL) and deoxyribonucleic acid (DNA) [169]. This formulation aims to enhance the delivery of therapeutic genes directly to cancer cells, improving the efficacy of the treatment while reducing potential side effects. The magnetic properties of the micelles may also facilitate targeted delivery and retention of the therapy within the tumor site [169].

Magnetic polymeric nanoformulations/hydrogels: polymeric nanoparticles are widely studied for biomedical applications because their compositions, structures, and properties can be controlled and adjusted [170, 171]. Polymeric nanoparticles' shape, size, surface charge, and functionalization can be easily fine-tuned, simultaneously allowing effective drug and MNP loading [170]. Researchers have developed an innovative polymeric magnetonanomaterial sensitive to pH and temperature. This nanomaterial is constructed using poly (D, L-lactic-co-glycolic acid) (PLGA), a biodegradable polymer widely used in medical applications. The nanomaterial features a shell containing superparamagnetic iron oxide nanoparticles (SPIONs), which enhance its magnetic properties and enable targeted delivery [171].

In addition to the SPIONs, the shell encapsulates two therapeutic agents: curcumin and 5-fluorouracil (5FU). Curcumin is known for its anti-inflammatory and anticancer properties, while 5FU is a commonly used chemotherapy drug that targets rapidly dividing cancer cells [172]. Figure 1.3 illustrates the detailed development of these MNPs. The combination of these components is designed to improve the effectiveness of cancer treatment by allowing for better targeting and controlled release of the drugs in response to the specific tumor microenvironment [172]. This advanced approach holds significant potential for enhancing cancer therapy, as it

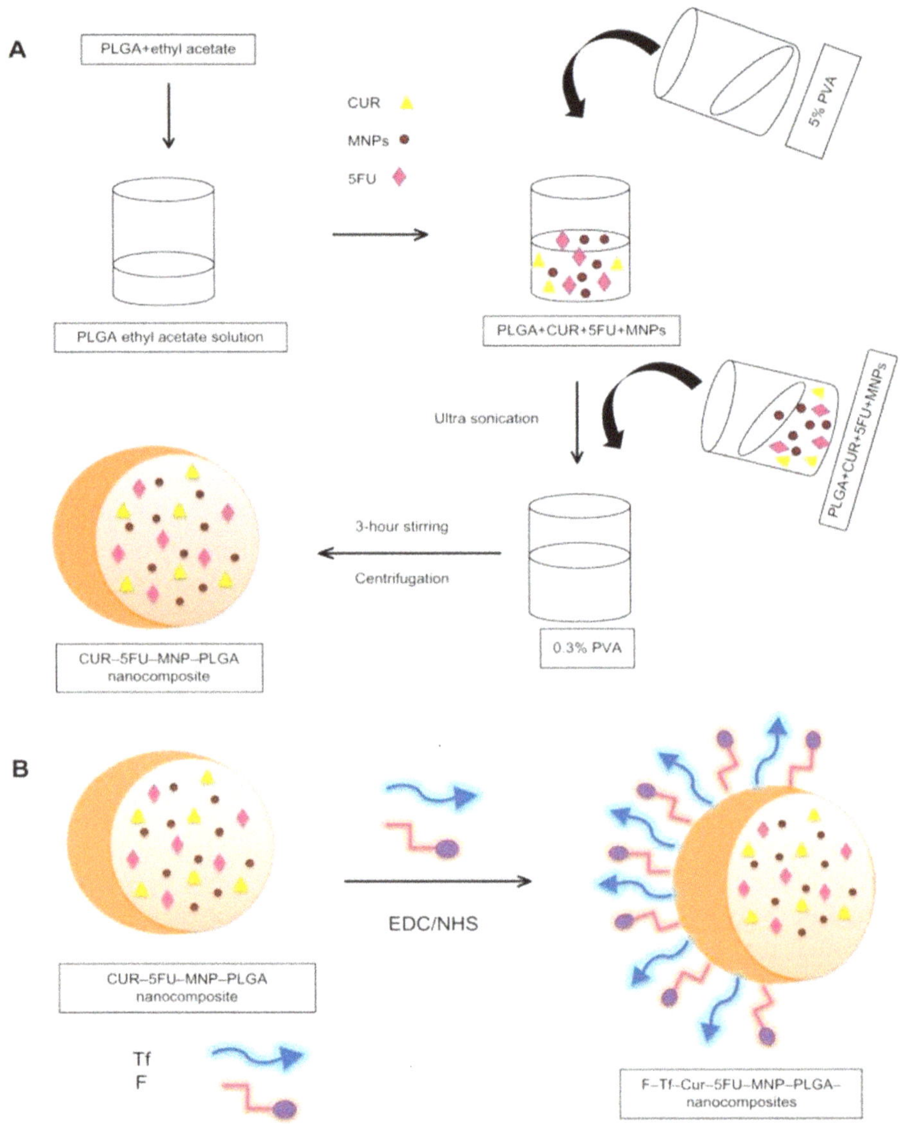

Figure 1.3. Schematic of the synthesis of dd–PLGA–MNPs and the biofunctionalization of NPs with F and Tf to form dt-dd–PLGA–MNPs. (A) Schematic of synthesis of dd–PLGA–MNPs; (B) biofunctionalization of NPs with F and Tf to form dt-dd–PLGA–MNPs. Reproduced with permissions from [172]. © 2013, The Author(s), CC BY-NC 3.0. Dove Medical Press Limited reprinted by permission of Informa UK Limited, trading as Taylor & Francis Ltd, http://www.tandfonline.com. Abbreviations: dd–PGLA–MNPs, double drug-loaded PGLA MNPs; dt–dd–PGLA–MNPs, double targeted double drug-loaded PGLA MNPs,

may increase the localized concentration of the drugs at the tumor site while minimizing side effects on healthy tissues. In a recent study, researchers developed a novel type of magnetic polymeric nanoparticle explicitly designed for the hyperthermic treatment of glioblastoma, a highly aggressive brain tumor. These nanoparticles are conjugated with Gly-Arg-Gly-Asp-Ser (GRGDS), a peptide known for its ability to target and bind to cancer cells, enhancing the delivery of therapeutic agents [173]. The nanoparticles are encapsulated in curcumin, a turmeric compound with anti-inflammatory and anticancer properties. This targeted approach aims to improve the efficacy of hyperthermia by ensuring that curcumin is delivered directly to the tumor site, where the heat generated by the nanoparticles can enhance the treatment's effectiveness while minimizing damage to surrounding healthy tissue [173].

Hydrogels are intricate materials constructed from a three-dimensional polymer network that retains water while maintaining insolubility due to their cross-linked structure [174]. They exhibit versatile properties, including elasticity, degradation rate, and swelling ratio, and these properties can be tailored by adjusting various parameters such as the type of polymer, block lengths, and cross-linker ratio [174]. Nanohydrogels are specifically employed as effective drug delivery systems, wherein drugs are entrapped within the polymer matrix and released via diffusion or matrix degradation. Furthermore, incorporating MNPs into the hydrogel matrix further expands their potential applications [175].

Folate-conjugated, doxorubicin-loaded, thermal-, and pH-responsive magnetic hydrogels have been developed as an innovative therapeutic approach for treating solid tumors [176]. These advanced hydrogels are designed to release the chemotherapeutic agent doxorubicin in response to specific thermal and pH conditions characteristic of tumor microenvironments. The hydrogels leverage the enhanced permeability and retention effect by incorporating folate conjugation, targeting cancer cells that overexpress folate receptors [176]. This magnetohydrogel system demonstrates a synergistic therapeutic effect by integrating chemotherapy with hyperthermia. External magnetic fields can heat the hydrogels locally, further enhancing drug release and cytotoxicity against tumor cells. This dual-action mechanism improves the treatment's efficacy and [176], Recently, researchers developed an innovative thermal-responsive magnetic hydrogel that incorporates β-cyclodextrin, iron oxide (Fe_3O_4), and the chemotherapy drug doxorubicin. This novel hydrogel is designed to enhance cancer treatment's effectiveness by combining chemotherapy and hyperthermic techniques. The β-cyclodextrin serves as a doxorubicin carrier, allowing for controlled drug release, while the Fe_3O_4 particles enable the hydrogel to respond to external magnetic fields and generate localized heat [177]. This dual approach aims to improve the targeting of cancer cells, minimize side effects, and increase the overall efficacy of treatment [177]. The existing research literature presents a diverse array of MNPs, categorized based on the materials from which they are constructed. These categories include metal-based nanoparticles, metal oxide nanoparticles, and polymer-based nanoparticles, each offering unique properties and applications. In the upcoming sections, we will examine some prominent examples of these nanoparticles, exploring their synthesis methods, structural characteristics, and potential applications in biomedicine, environmental remediation, and data storage. This comprehensive analysis will highlight the advancements and challenges associated with each type of MNP.

1.2 Applications of magnetic nanoparticles in cancer theranostics

Recently, MNPs have been widely used for biomedical applications because of their biocompatibility and low toxicity [27, 178]. Further, MNPs have made tremendous advancements in cancer theranostics, some of which have even reached clinical trials [179]. The synthesis process can easily tune the MNP properties. They can be designed according to the needs of theranostic applications, as these properties determine the biodistribution and pharmacokinetics of the nanoparticles [180]. These MNPs can act as magnetically guided delivery agents and theranostic agents [181]. In addition, these MNPs can also be used as contrast agents in MRI. This section discusses some of the important biomedical applications of MNPs in cancer theranostics [179].

Magnetically guided drug delivery has become popular recently. In this approach, an external magnetic field is used to control the movement of MNPs [182]. The drug-loaded MNPs can be transported to the target site and are easily eliminated after complete treatment. This concept reduces toxicity to normal cells and increases the drug's effect at the target site [182]. The MNPs are usually coated with other materials, such as polymers, to increase their aqueous solubility and prevent agglomeration. Silica, carbon, polymers, surfactants, and proteins are the most frequently used coating materials, offering a wide range of protective and functional benefits. Once the drug-loaded MNPs are injected into the bloodstream, they can be guided to the target site using an external magnetic field. As a result, these MNPs can easily accumulate at tumor sites due to the EPR effect [178].

For instance, Chorny *et al* successfully synthesized iron-oxide-based MNPs coated with calcium oleate and loaded with two important enzymes: superoxide dismutase (SOD) and catalase (CAT). These MNPs were designed to enhance therapeutic efficacy by facilitating targeted delivery and reducing oxidative stress in biological systems [183]. The researchers investigated the effectiveness of these MNPs under two conditions: with and without the application of an external magnetic field. Their findings revealed that when the MNPs were exposed to a magnetic field for 10 min, there was a remarkable increase in the internalization of the nanoparticles into target cells compared to the situation without the magnetic field. This significant enhancement in MNP uptake suggests that an external magnetic field can be crucial in improving the delivery and therapeutic potential of enzyme-loaded MNPs [183]. Similarly, researchers created iron oxide nanoparticles (IONPs) coated with starch to enhance their stability and biocompatibility [184]. They conducted a series of experiments to assess the effectiveness of these nanoparticles in targeting and treating breast cancer cells. The study was designed to evaluate the response of the cancer cells under two different conditions: one where external magnetic fields were applied and another where no external fields were present. This investigation aimed to determine how the presence of these fields might influence the therapeutic potential of starch-coated IONPs in breast cancer treatment [184].

A recent study highlighted the effectiveness of citrate-functionalized magnetite nanoparticles, which demonstrated remarkable colloidal stability. Researchers employed sucrose as a cryoprotectant, facilitating these nanoparticles' long-term preservation by forming a well-defined clustered shell nanostructure. This innovative structure, composed of citrate–magnetite and chitosan, was particularly useful in targeted antitumor therapies. This study emphasized the importance of this unique citrate–magnetite/chitosan cluster–shell nanoparticle in enhancing the efficacy of hyperthermic treatment for cancer [185]. By utilizing a systemic dual magneto–photothermal therapy approach, this nanostructure precisely targeted tumor cells while simultaneously elevating local temperatures to induce cell death. This methodological advancement represents a promising direction in cancer treatment, combining nanotechnology with thermal therapy for better therapeutic outcomes [185].

In another recent study, researchers made significant advancements by developing MNPs coated with dextran and carboxymethyl dextran [186]. These innovative Fe_3O_4 MNPs showed great potential in accurately labeling breast cancer cells. Using these coated nanoparticles enhances the targeting and visualization of cancer cells, which could lead to improved diagnostic and therapeutic strategies in the fight against breast cancer [186]. This breakthrough could pave the way for more effective treatments and monitoring techniques in oncology [186]. Iqbal *et al* conducted research on the development of cobalt iron oxide ($CoFe_2O_4$) MNPs coated with silicon dioxide (SiO_2) [187]. This innovative approach aims to leverage the properties of these nanoparticles for potential applications in cancer treatment, specifically through a technique known as magnetic hyperthermia [187]. In this method, the nanoparticles can be subjected to an alternating magnetic field, which generates localized heat, effectively targeting and destroying cancer cells while minimizing damage to surrounding healthy tissue. The SiO_2 coating enhances the biocompatibility and stability of the $CoFe_2O_4$ nanoparticles, further improving their efficacy in a clinical setting [187].

MNPs are a promising technology that facilitates targeted drug delivery to specific sites within the body by utilizing magnetic targeting techniques [188]. This approach allows for precise control over the location and concentration of therapeutic agents, potentially enhancing treatment efficacy while minimizing side effects. Furthermore, the effectiveness of these nanoformulations, which combine MNPs with various drugs, can be monitored through MRI. This is possible because MNPs, especially those made from iron oxide, act as excellent contrast agents, enabling more precise imaging and tracking of the nanoparticles within biological systems [189]. MNPs offer a wide array of potential applications in biomedicine, making them an exciting area of research. One of the most intriguing applications is magnetic hyperthermia, a treatment method that involves heating tumor cells using magnetic fields to destroy cancerous tissue while selectively preserving surrounding healthy cells [27]. This technique has gained considerable attention within the scientific community and has prompted significant research efforts to optimize its effectiveness and understand its mechanisms [27]. The diverse capabilities of MNPs highlight their significant potential to transform the landscape of targeted therapies. By enabling precise delivery of therapeutic agents directly to affected cells or tissues, MNPs can effectively minimize side effects associated with traditional treatments. This targeted approach enhances treatment efficacy and improves patient outcomes across various medical conditions, including cancer, cardiovascular diseases, and neurological disorders. As research advances, the integration of MNPs into clinical applications promises to revolutionize treatment strategies and provide innovative solutions for needy patients.

References

[1] Visakh P 2024 Recent progress in nanobiotechnology: modern techniques in biomedical applications: state-of-the-art and new challenges *Recent Progress in Nanobiotechnology: Modern Techniques in Biomedical Applications* (Singapore: Springer) pp 1–20

[2] Sobha K, Surendranath K, Meena V, Jwala K, Swetha N and Latha K 2010 Emerging trends in nanobiotechnology *Biotechnol. Mol. Biol. Rev.* **4** 5FF052811265

[3] Sharaf M and Issa S A S 2025 Applications of nanobiotechnology in the field of exercise physiology *Int. Sports Sci. Alex. J.* **7** 1–7

[4] Liu X, Liu S, Jin X, Liu H, Sun K, Wang X, Li M, Wang P, Chang Y and Wang T 2024 An encounter between metal ions and natural products: natural products-coordinated metal ions for the diagnosis and treatment of tumors *J. Nanobiotechnol.* **22** 726

[5] Fathi-karkan S, Easwaran E C, Kharaba Z, Rahdar A and Pandey S 2024 Unlocking mysteries: the cutting-edge fusion of nanotechnology and forensic science *BioNanoScience* **14** 3572–98

[6] Kumar P, Thakur N, Kumar K, Kumar S, Dutt A, Thakur V K, Gutiérrez-Rodelo C, Thakur P, Navarrete A and Thakur N 2024 Catalyzing innovation: exploring iron oxide nanoparticles-origins, advancements, and future application horizons *Coord. Chem. Rev.* **507** 215750

[7] Singh A and Sahoo S K 2014 Magnetic nanoparticles: a novel platform for cancer theranostics *Drug Discov. Today* **19** 474–81

[8] Comanescu C 2023 Recent advances in surface functionalization of magnetic nanoparticles *Coatings* **13** 1772

[9] Farinha P D F 2021 Magnetic Nanoparticles in Diagnostics: A Review of Recent Advances *PQDT-Global* 31708149

[10] Farinha P, Coelho J M, Reis C P and Gaspar M M 2021 A comprehensive updated review on magnetic nanoparticles in diagnostics *Nanomaterials* **11** 3432

[11] Rastogi A, Yadav K, Mishra A, Singh M S, Chaudhary S, Manohar R and Parmar A S 2022 Early diagnosis of lung cancer using magnetic nanoparticles-integrated systems *Nanotechnol. Rev.* **11** 544–74

[12] Andoh V, Ocansey D K W, Naveed H, Wang N, Chen L, Chen K and Mao F 2024 The advancing role of nanocomposites in cancer diagnosis and treatment *Int. J. Nanomed.* **19** 6099–126

[13] Anik M I, Hossain M K, Hossain I, Mahfuz A, Rahman M T and Ahmed I 2021 Recent progress of magnetic nanoparticles in biomedical applications: a review *Nano Select* **2** 1146–86

[14] Cardoso V F, Francesko A, Ribeiro C, Bañobre-López M, Martins P and Lanceros-Mendez S 2018 Advances in magnetic nanoparticles for biomedical applications *Adv. Healthc. Mater.* **7** 1700845

[15] Bohara R A, Thorat N D and Pawar S H 2016 Role of functionalization: strategies to explore potential nano-bio applications of magnetic nanoparticles *RSC Adv.* **6** 43989–4012

[16] Negi R, Yadav R, Upadhye V J, Jain B and Berdimurodov E 2025 Design and movements of drug in human metabolism by multifunctional magnetic nanoparticles *Multifunctional Magnetic Nanoparticles in Therapy, Biology, and Pharmacy* (Boca Raton, FL: CRC Press) pp 92–113

[17] Zhu S, Xu L, Zhang Y, Zheng Z, Lang Z, Zhang Q, Gao J, Ye M and Xu R X 2024 Magnetically controlled strategies for enhanced tissue vascularization *Adv. Funct. Mater.* **34** 2401856
[18] Mishra S and Yadav M D 2024 Magnetic nanoparticles: a comprehensive review from synthesis to biomedical frontiers *Langmuir* **40** 17239–69
[19] Moulahoum H, Ghorbanizamani F, Tok K and Zihnioglu F 2024 Introduction to magnetic nanosystems: classifications, structure, properties, biological interactions, and diagnostic applications *Functionalized Magnetic Nanosystems for Diagnostic Tools and Devices* (Amsterdam: Elsevier) pp 1–41
[20] Manescu V, Paltanea G, Antoniac I and Vasilescu M 2021 Magnetic nanoparticles used in oncology *Materials* **14** 5948
[21] Selim M M, El-Safty S, Tounsi A and Shenashen M 2024 A review of magnetic nanoparticles used in nanomedicine *APL Mater.* **12** 010601
[22] Fang C and Zhang M 2009 Multifunctional magnetic nanoparticles for medical imaging applications *J. Mater. Chem.* **19** 6258–66
[23] Mittal A, Roy I and Gandhi S 2022 Magnetic nanoparticles: an overview for biomedical applications *Magnetochemistry* **8** 107
[24] AboGabal R, Shokeir D and Oraby A 2023 Design and synthesis of biologically inspired biocompatible various polymeric magnetic nanoparticles for imaging and biomedical applications *Nano-Struct. Nano-Objects* **36** 101048
[25] Lee H, Shin T-H, Cheon J and Weissleder R 2015 Recent developments in magnetic diagnostic systems *Chem. Rev.* **115** 10690–724
[26] Berdimurodov E, Hussain C M and Tüzün B 2024 *Multifunctional Magnetic Nanoparticles in Therapy, Biology, and Pharmacy: Synthesis, Fundamentals and Applications* (Boca Raton, FL: CRC Press)
[27] Materón E M, Miyazaki C M, Carr O, Joshi N, Picciani P H, Dalmaschio C J, Davis F and Shimizu F M 2021 Magnetic nanoparticles in biomedical applications: a review *Appl. Surf. Sci. Adv.* **6** 100163
[28] Yang H Y, Li Y and Lee D S 2018 Multifunctional and stimuli-responsive magnetic nanoparticle-based delivery systems for biomedical applications *Adv. Therap.* **1** 1800011
[29] Khan S, Ahmad V, Hassan Baig M, Amjad Kamal M, Ahmad S, Rai M, Muhammad Zafar Iqbal A, Mushtaq G and Sajid Khan M 2015 Magnetic nanoparticles: properties, synthesis and biomedical applications *Curr. Drug Metab.* **16** 685–704
[30] Ali A, Shah T, Ullah R, Zhou P, Guo M, Ovais M, Tan Z and Rui Y 2021 Review on recent progress in magnetic nanoparticles: synthesis, characterization, and diverse applications *Front. Chem.* **9** 629054
[31] Kianfar E 2021 Magnetic nanoparticles in targeted drug delivery: a review *J. Supercond. Nov. Magn.* **34** 1709–35
[32] Sun C, Lee J S and Zhang M 2008 Magnetic nanoparticles in MR imaging and drug delivery *Adv. Drug Deliv. Rev.* **60** 1252–65
[33] Sheha R R 2024 Magnetic composites: fundamentals, synthesis, and applications *Magnetic Nanoparticles and Polymer Nanocomposites* (Amsterdam: Elsevier) pp 303–71
[34] Spoială A, Ilie C-I, Crăciun L N, Ficai D, Ficai A and Andronescu E 2021 Magnetite-silica core/shell nanostructures: from surface functionalization towards biomedical applications—a review *Appl. Sci.* **11** 11075

[35] Yoon T J, Yu K N, Kim E, Kim J S, Kim B G, Yun S H, Sohn B H, Cho M H, Lee J K and Park S B 2006 Specific targeting, cell sorting, and bioimaging with smart magnetic silica core–shell nanomaterials *small* **2** 209–15

[36] Sun Z, Zhou X, Luo W, Yue Q, Zhang Y, Cheng X, Li W, Kong B, Deng Y and Zhao D 2016 Interfacial engineering of magnetic particles with porous shells: Towards magnetic core–porous shell microparticles *Nano Today* **11** 464–82

[37] Lu A H, Salabas E e L and Schüth F 2007 Magnetic nanoparticles: synthesis, protection, functionalization, and application *Angew. Chem. Int. Ed.* **46** 1222–44

[38] Tran H-V, Ngo N M, Medhi R, Srinoi P, Liu T, Rittikulsittichai S and Lee T R 2022 Multifunctional iron oxide magnetic nanoparticles for biomedical applications: a review *Materials* **15** 503

[39] Shubayev V I, Pisanic T R II and Jin S 2009 Magnetic nanoparticles for theragnostics *Adv. Drug Deliv. Rev.* **61** 467–77

[40] Issa B, Obaidat I M, Albiss B A and Haik Y 2013 Magnetic nanoparticles: surface effects and properties related to biomedicine applications *Int. J. Mol. Sci.* **14** 21266–305

[41] Oubaaqa M, Rbaa M and Berdimurodov E 2025 Multifunctional magnetic nanoparticles in nanotoxicology *Multifunctional Magnetic Nanoparticles in Therapy, Biology, and Pharmacy* (Boca Raton, FL: CRC Press) pp 242–56

[42] Sun W, Chai X, Zhang Y, Yu T, Wang Y, Zhao W, Liu Y, Yin D and Zhang C 2024 Combination using magnetic iron oxide nanoparticles and magnetic field for cancer therapy *Chem. Rec.* **24** e202400179

[43] Rezaei B, Yari P, Sanders S M, Wang H, Chugh V K, Liang S, Mostufa S, Xu K, Wang J P and Gómez-Pastora J 2024 Magnetic nanoparticles: a review on synthesis, characterization, functionalization, and biomedical applications *Small* **20** 2304848

[44] Singh R, Yadav D, Ingole P G and Ahn Y-H 2024 Magnetic engineering nanoparticles: versatile tools revolutionizing biomedical applications *Biomater. Adv.* **163** 213948

[45] Araújo E, Carneiro S, Neto D, Freire T, Costa V, Freire R, Fechine L, Clemente C, Denardin J and Dos Santos J 2024 Advances in surface design and biomedical applications of magnetic nanoparticles *Adv. Colloid Interface Sci.* **328** 103166

[46] Shakeri-Zadeh A and Bulte J W 2024 Imaging-guided precision hyperthermia with magnetic nanoparticles *Nat. Rev. Bioeng.* **3** 245–60

[47] Sharma S, Sharma H and Sharma R 2024 A review on functionalization and potential application spectrum of magnetic nanoparticles (MNPs) based systems *Chem. Inorgan. Mater.* **2** 100035

[48] Stiufiuc G F and Stiufiuc R I 2024 Magnetic nanoparticles: synthesis, characterization, and their use in biomedical field *Appl. Sci.* **14** 1623

[49] Hong J, Wang L, Zheng Q, Cai C, Yang X and Liao Z 2024 The recent applications of magnetic nanoparticles in biomedical fields *Materials* **17** 2870

[50] Al-Thani A N, Jan A G, Abbas M, Geetha M and Sadasivuni K K 2024 Nanoparticles in cancer theragnostic and drug delivery: a comprehensive review *Life Sci.* **352** 122899

[51] Gobbo O L, Sjaastad K, Radomski M W, Volkov Y and Prina-Mello A 2015 Magnetic nanoparticles in cancer theranostics *Theranostics* **5** 1249

[52] Huang J, Li Y, Orza A, Lu Q, Guo P, Wang L, Yang L and Mao H 2016 Magnetic nanoparticle facilitated drug delivery for cancer therapy with targeted and image-guided approaches *Adv. Funct. Mater.* **26** 3818–36

[53] Veiseh O, Gunn J W and Zhang M 2010 Design and fabrication of magnetic nanoparticles for targeted drug delivery and imaging *Adv. Drug Deliv. Rev.* **62** 284–304
[54] Wang M, Jin L, Hang-Mei Leung P, Wang-Ngai Chow F, Zhao X, Chen H, Pan W, Liu H and Li S 2024 Advancements in magnetic nanoparticle-based biosensors for point-of-care testing *Front. Bioeng. Biotechnol.* **12** 1393789
[55] Martins P M, Lima A C, Ribeiro S, Lanceros-Mendez S and Martins P 2021 Magnetic nanoparticles for biomedical applications: from the soul of the earth to the deep history of ourselves *ACS Appl. Bio Mater.* **4** 5839–70
[56] Malehmir S, Esmaili M A, Khaksary Mahabady M, Sobhani-Nasab A, Atapour A, Ganjali M R, Ghasemi A and Moradi Hasan-Abad A 2023 A review: hemocompatibility of magnetic nanoparticles and their regenerative medicine, cancer therapy, drug delivery, and bioimaging applications *Front. Chem.* **11** 1249134
[57] Chandrakala V, Aruna V and Angajala G 2022 Review on metal nanoparticles as nanocarriers: current challenges and perspectives in drug delivery systems *Emerg. Mater.* **5** 1593–615
[58] Wani S U D, Ali M, Masoodi M H, Khan N A, Zargar M I, Hassan R, Mir S A, Gautam S P, Gangadharappa H and Osmani R A M 2022 A review on nanoparticles categorization, characterization and applications in drug delivery systems *Vib. Spectrosc.* **121** 103407
[59] Karami M H, Abdouss M and Maleki B 2024 The state of the art metal nanoparticles in drug delivery systems: a comprehensive review *Nanomed. J.* **11** 222–49
[60] Gavilán H, Avugadda S K, Fernández-Cabada T, Soni N, Cassani M, Mai B T, Chantrell R and Pellegrino T 2021 Magnetic nanoparticles and clusters for magnetic hyperthermia: optimizing their heat performance and developing combinatorial therapies to tackle cancer *Chem. Soc. Rev.* **50** 11614–67
[61] Li X, Li W, Wang M and Liao Z 2021 Magnetic nanoparticles for cancer theranostics: advances and prospects *J. Control. Release* **335** 437–48
[62] Farzin A, Etesami S A, Quint J, Memic A and Tamayol A 2020 Magnetic nanoparticles in cancer therapy and diagnosis *Adv. Healthc. Mater.* **9** 1901058
[63] Fakhradini S S, Mosharaf-Dehkordi M and Ahmadikia H 2024 Enhancing liver cancer treatment: exploring the frequency effects of magnetic nanoparticles for heat-based tumor therapy with microwaves *Int. J. Therm. Sci.* **203** 109154
[64] Kwizera E A, Stewart S, Mahmud M M and He X 2022 Magnetic nanoparticle-mediated heating for biomedical applications *J. Heat Transfer* **144** 030801
[65] Chang M, Hou Z, Wang M, Li C and Lin J 2021 Recent advances in hyperthermia therapy-based synergistic immunotherapy *Adv. Mater.* **33** 2004788
[66] Kumar C S and Mohammad F 2011 Magnetic nanomaterials for hyperthermia-based therapy and controlled drug delivery *Adv. Drug Deliv. Rev.* **63** 789–808
[67] Chen W H, Luo G F and Zhang X Z 2019 Recent advances in subcellular targeted cancer therapy based on functional materials *Adv. Mater.* **31** 1802725
[68] Assa F, Jafarizadeh-Malmiri H, Ajamein H, Vaghari H, Anarjan N, Ahmadi O and Berenjian A 2017 Chitosan magnetic nanoparticles for drug delivery systems *Crit. Rev. Biotechnol.* **37** 492–509
[69] Zhuo Y, Zhao Y-G and Zhang Y 2024 Enhancing drug solubility, bioavailability, and targeted therapeutic applications through magnetic nanoparticles *Molecules* **29** 4854
[70] Spoială A, Ilie C-I, Motelica L, Ficai D, Semenescu A, Oprea O-C and Ficai A 2023 Smart magnetic drug delivery systems for the treatment of cancer *Nanomaterials* **13** 876

[71] Albinali K E, Zagho M M, Deng Y and Elzatahry A A 2019 A perspective on magnetic core–shell carriers for responsive and targeted drug delivery systems *Int. J. Nanomed.* **14** 1707–23

[72] Sensenig R, Sapir Y, MacDonald C, Cohen S and Polyak B 2012 Magnetic nanoparticle-based approaches to locally target therapy and enhance tissue regeneration *in vivo Nanomedicine* **7** 1425–42

[73] Dilnawaz F and Sahoo S K 2015 Therapeutic approaches of magnetic nanoparticles for the central nervous system *Drug Discov. Today* **20** 1256–64

[74] SV S, Augustine D, Hosmani J, Pagnoni F, Reda R, Testarelli L and Patil S 2024 Nanoparticle-based biomolecules in cancer diagnosis, therapy, drug delivery and prognosis *Front. Dental Med.* **5** 1482166

[75] Abaei S, Tarighatnia A, Mesbahi A and Aghanejad A 2024 Antibody conjugates as CT/MRI theranostics for diagnosis of cancers: a review of recent trends and advances *Sens. Diag.* **3** 1428–41

[76] Bushra R, Ahmad M, Alam K, Seidi F, Shakeel S, Song J, Jin Y and Xiao H 2024 Recent advances in magnetic nanoparticles: key applications, environmental insights, and future strategies *Sustain. Mater. Technol.* **40** e00985

[77] Najdian A, Beiki D, Abbasi M, Gholamrezanezhad A, Ahmadzadehfar H, Amani A M, Ardestani M S and Assadi M 2024 Exploring innovative strides in radiolabeled nano-particle progress for multimodality cancer imaging and theranostic applications *Cancer Imag.* **24** 127

[78] Kul İ B, Tüzün G, Tüzün B, Berdimurodov E and Rbaa M 2025 Multifunctional magnetic nanoparticles in the separation and detection of biological molecules: proteins, enzymes, and nucleic acid *Multifunctional Magnetic Nanoparticles in Therapy, Biology, and Pharmacy* (Boca Raton, FL: CRC Press) pp 155–70

[79] Lee Y-Y, Sriram B, Wang S-F, Kogularasu S and Chang-Chien G-P 2024 Advanced nanomaterial-based biosensors for N-terminal pro-brain natriuretic peptide biomarker detection: progress and future challenges in cardiovascular disease diagnostics *Nanomaterials* **14** 153

[80] Tripathi N K, Trivedi R K, Sambamoorthy U, Mishra S, Dharmalingam S, Bagde M P, Aijaz M and Verma G 2024 Biomedical applications of magnetic nanoparticles: current trends and future perspectives *Biochem. Cell. Arch.* **24** 413–24

[81] Eivazzadeh-Keihan R, Bahreinizad H, Amiri Z, Aliabadi H A M, Salimi-Bani M, Nakisa A, Davoodi F, Tahmasebi B, Ahmadpour F and Radinekiyan F 2021 Functionalized magnetic nanoparticles for the separation and purification of proteins and peptides *TrAC, Trends Anal. Chem.* **141** 116291

[82] Nekounam H, Babaei M, Kisomi M F, Pourkhodadad S, Mahmoodi N, Nazbar A, Hasanzadeh E, Zarei M and Faridi-Majidi R 2022 Application of functional magnetic nanoparticles for separation of target materials: a review *Curr. Nanosci.* **18** 554–70

[83] Zhou Q, Zhang L and Wu H 2017 Nanomaterials for cancer therapies *Nanotechnol. Rev.* **6** 473–96

[84] Vallabani N V, Singh S and Karakoti A S 2019 Magnetic nanoparticles: current trends and future aspects in diagnostics and nanomedicine *Curr. Drug Metab.* **20** 457–72

[85] Santos L F, Silva A S and Mano J F 2023 Magnetic-based strategies for regenerative medicine and tissue engineering *Adv. Healthc. Mater.* **12** 2300605

[86] Faraji M 2016 Recent analytical applications of magnetic nanoparticles *Nanochem. Res.* **1** 264–90

[87] Rios A, Zougagh M and Bouri M 2013 Magnetic (nano) materials as an useful tool for sample preparation in analytical methods. A review *Anal. Methods* **5** 4558–73

[88] He J, Huang M, Wang D, Zhang Z and Li G 2014 Magnetic separation techniques in sample preparation for biological analysis: a review *J. Pharm. Biomed. Anal.* **101** 84–101

[89] Xiao F, Li W and Xu H 2022 Advances in magnetic nanoparticles for the separation of foodborne pathogens: recognition, separation strategy, and application *Compr. Rev. Food Sci. Food Saf.* **21** 4478–504

[90] Tang C, He Z, Liu H, Xu Y, Huang H, Yang G, Xiao Z, Li S, Liu H and Deng Y 2020 Application of magnetic nanoparticles in nucleic acid detection *J. Nanobiotechnol.* **18** 1–19

[91] Antwi-Baah R, Wang Y, Chen X and Yu K 2022 Metal-based nanoparticle magnetic resonance imaging contrast agents: classifications, issues, and countermeasures toward their clinical translation *Adv. Mater. Interfaces* **9** 2101710

[92] Aram E, Moeni M, Abedizadeh R, Sabour D, Sadeghi-Abandansari H, Gardy J and Hassanpour A 2022 Smart and multi-functional magnetic nanoparticles for cancer treatment applications: clinical challenges and future prospects *Nanomaterials* **12** 3567

[93] Ferreira M, Sousa J, Pais A and Vitorino C 2020 The role of magnetic nanoparticles in cancer nanotheranostics *Materials* **13** 266

[94] Khizar S, Elkalla E, Zine N, Jaffrezic-Renault N, Errachid A and Elaissari A 2023 Magnetic nanoparticles: multifunctional tool for cancer therapy *Exp. Opinion Drug Deliv.* **20** 189–204

[95] Ko M J, Hong H, Choi H, Kang H and Kim D H 2022 Multifunctional magnetic nanoparticles for dynamic imaging and therapy *Adv. NanoBiomed Res.* **2** 2200053

[96] Szwed M and Marczak A 2024 Application of nanoparticles for magnetic hyperthermia for cancer treatment—the current state of knowledge *Cancers* **16** 1156

[97] Egea-Benavente D, Ovejero J G, Morales M d P and Barber D F 2021 Understanding MNPs behaviour in response to AMF in biological milieus and the effects at the cellular level: Implications for a rational design that drives magnetic hyperthermia therapy toward clinical implementation *Cancers* **13** 4583

[98] Ali A, Zafar H, Zia M, ul Haq I, Phull A R, Ali J S and Hussain A 2016 Synthesis, characterization, applications, and challenges of iron oxide nanoparticles *Nanotechnol. Sci. Appl.* **9** 49–67

[99] Zhu N, Ji H, Yu P, Niu J, Farooq M, Akram M W, Udego I, Li H and Niu X 2018 Surface modification of magnetic iron oxide nanoparticles *Nanomaterials* **8** 810

[100] Ogbezode J E, Ezealigo U S, Bello A, Anye V C and Onwualu A P 2023 A narrative review of the synthesis, characterization, and applications of iron oxide nanoparticles *Discov. Nano* **18** 125

[101] Tejashwini D, Harini H, Nagaswarupa H, Naik R, Deshmukh V and Basavaraju N 2023 An in-depth exploration of eco-friendly synthesis methods for metal oxide nanoparticles and their role in photocatalysis for industrial dye degradation *Chem. Phys. Impact* **7** 100355

[102] Obisesan O S, Ajiboye T O, Mhlanga S D and Mufhandu H T 2023 Biomedical applications of biodegradable polycaprolactone-functionalized magnetic iron oxides nanoparticles and their polymer nanocomposites *Colloids Surf.*, B **227** 113342

[103] Yang Y, Liu Y, Song L, Cui X, Zhou J, Jin G, Boccaccini A R and Virtanen S 2023 Iron oxide nanoparticle-based nanocomposites in biomedical application *Trends Biotechnol.* **41** 1471–87

[104] Vasić K, Knez Ž and Leitgeb M 2024 Multifunctional iron oxide nanoparticles as promising magnetic biomaterials in drug delivery: a review *J. Funct. Biomater.* **15** 227
[105] Alzoubi F, Noqta O A, AlZoubi T, AlJabaly H, Alkhateeb H, Alqadi M and Makhadmeh G 2023 Exploring the impact of pH on the properties of citric acid-coated iron oxide nanoparticles as high-performance T2 contrast agent for MRI applications *Res. Eng.* **18** 101206
[106] Truong T T, Mondal S, Doan V H M, Tak S, Choi J, Oh H, Nguyen T D, Misra M, Lee B and Oh J 2024 Precision-engineered metal and metal-oxide nanoparticles for biomedical imaging and healthcare applications *Adv. Colloid Interface Sci.* **332** 103263
[107] Gupta I, Sirohi S and Roy K 2023 Strategies for functionalization of magnetic nanoparticles for biomedical applications *Mater. Today Proc.* **72** 2757–67
[108] Chikhaliwala P and Chandra S 2023 Recent status of the current clinical trials going on for superparamagnetic materials *Superparamagnetic Materials for Cancer Medicine* (Berlin: Springer) pp 243–68
[109] Lapusan R, Borlan R and Focsan M 2024 Advancing MRI with magnetic nanoparticles: a comprehensive review of translational research and clinical trials *Nanoscale Adv.* **6** 2234–59
[110] Abdelkawi A, Slim A, Zinoune Z and Pathak Y 2023 Surface modification of metallic nanoparticles for targeting drugs *Coatings* **13** 1660
[111] Rayhan M A, Hossen M S, Niloy M S, Bhuiyan M H, Paul S and Shakil M S 2021 Biopolymer and biomaterial conjugated Iron oxide nanomaterials as prostate cancer theranostic agents: a comprehensive review *Symmetry* **13** 974
[112] Mahmoudi K, Bouras A, Bozec D, Ivkov R and Hadjipanayis C 2018 Magnetic hyperthermia therapy for the treatment of glioblastoma: a review of the therapy's history, efficacy and application in humans *Int. J. Hyperth.* **34** 1316–28
[113] Bayda S, Adeel M, Tuccinardi T, Cordani M and Rizzolio F 2019 The history of nanoscience and nanotechnology: from chemical-physical applications to nanomedicine *Molecules* **25** 112
[114] Kumar T, Pandey R K, Kumar R, Sudheep C V, Sreelakshmi S, Awasthi S, Vandana and Singhal R 2024 Historical perspective of nanotechnology and functionalized nanomaterials *Functionalized Nanomaterials Based Supercapacitor: Design, Performance and Industrial Applications* ed C M Hussain and M B Ahamed (Singapore: Springer Nature) pp 3–24
[115] Heiligtag F J and Niederberger M 2013 The fascinating world of nanoparticle research *Mater. Today* **16** 262–71
[116] Ball P 2003 Renaissance potters were nanotechnologists *Nature* https://doi.org/10.1038/news030623-17
[117] Sharma N 2020 *Self-organization of Silver Nanoparticles with Femtosecond Laser in TiO_2 Matrix: Applications to Plasmonic Colours, Multiple Hidden Images and Colour Image-Multiplexing* (Lyon: Université de Lyon) https://hal.science/tel-03117138v1
[118] Jana J, Ganguly M and Pal T 2016 Enlightening surface plasmon resonance effect of metal nanoparticles for practical spectroscopic application *RSC Adv.* **6** 86174–211
[119] Sanders W 2018 *Basic Principles of Nanotechnology* (Boca Raton, FL: CRC Press)
[120] Michos F I, Chronis A G, Garoufalis C S and Sigalas M M 2024 Optical properties of Cu, Ag, and Au nanoparticles with different sizes and shapes *Appl. Res.* **3** e202300101
[121] Polte J 2015 Fundamental growth principles of colloidal metal nanoparticles—a new perspective *CrystEngComm* **17** 6809–30

[122] Edwards P P and Thomas J M 2007 Gold in a metallic divided state—from faraday to present-day nanoscience *Angew. Chem. Int. Ed.* **46** 5480–6

[123] Talapin D V and Shevchenko E V 2016 Introduction: nanoparticle chemistry *Chem. Rev.* **116** 10343–5

[124] Baratoff A 1986 Nobel prizes development of scanning tunnelling microscopy *Europhys. News* **17** 141–4

[125] Bian K, Gerber C, Heinrich A J, Müller D J, Scheuring S and Jiang Y 2021 Scanning probe microscopy *Nat. Rev. Methods Primers* **1** 36

[126] Hansma P K, Elings V B, Marti O and Bracker C E 1988 Scanning tunneling microscopy and atomic force microscopy: application to biology and technology *Science* **242** 209–16

[127] Borode A O, Tshephe T S, Akinwamide S O and Olubambi P A 2025 Nanotechnology characterization: emerging techniques for accurate and reliable nanostructural analysis *Smart Nanomaterials for Environmental Applications* ed O O Ayeleru, A O Idris, S Pandey and P A Olubambi (Amsterdam: Elsevier) ch 3 pp 57–91

[128] Capek I 2019 *Nanocomposite Structures and Dispersions* 2nd edn (Amsterdam: Elsevier)

[129] Wang J, Zhao W, Zhang Z, Liu X, Xie T, Wang L, Xue Y and Zhang Y 2024 A journey of challenges and victories: a bibliometric worldview of nanomedicine since the 21st century *Adv. Mater.* **36** 2308915

[130] Kaur L, Sohal H S, Kaur M, Malhi D S and Garg S 2020 A mini-review on nano technology in the tumour targeting strategies: drug delivery to cancer cells *Anti-Cancer Agents Med. Chem.* **20** 2012–24

[131] Bayda S, Adeel M, Tuccinardi T, Cordani M and Rizzolio F 2020 The history of nanoscience and nanotechnology: from chemical–physical applications to nanomedicine *Molecules* **25** 112

[132] Banerjee R, Katsenovich Y, Lagos L, McIintosh M, Zhang X and Li C-Z 2010 Nanomedicine: magnetic nanoparticles and their biomedical applications *Curr. Med. Chem.* **17** 3120–41

[133] Shabestari Khiabani S, Farshbaf M, Akbarzadeh A and Davaran S 2017 Magnetic nanoparticles: preparation methods, applications in cancer diagnosis and cancer therapy *Artif. Cells, Nanomed., Biotechnol.* **45** 6–17

[134] Mohapatra M and Anand S 2010 Synthesis and applications of nano-structured iron oxides/hydroxides—a review *Int. J. Eng., Sci. Technol.* **2** 127–46

[135] Kefeni K K, Mamba B B and Msagati T A 2017 Application of spinel ferrite nanoparticles in water and wastewater treatment: a review *Sep. Purif. Technol.* **188** 399–422

[136] Dippong T, Levei E A and Cadar O 2021 Recent advances in synthesis and applications of MFe(2)O(4) (M = Co, Cu, Mn, Ni, Zn) nanoparticles *Nanomaterials (Basel)* **11** 1560

[137] Salih S J and Mahmood W M 2023 Review on magnetic spinel ferrite (MFe_2O_4) nanoparticles: from synthesis to application *Heliyon* **9** e16601

[138] Tadic M, Kralj S, Jagodic M, Hanzel D and Makovec D 2014 Magnetic properties of novel superparamagnetic iron oxide nanoclusters and their peculiarity under annealing treatment *Appl. Surf. Sci.* **322** 255–64

[139] Reddy L H, Arias J L, Nicolas J and Couvreur P 2012 Magnetic nanoparticles: design and characterization, toxicity and biocompatibility, pharmaceutical and biomedical applications *Chem. Rev.* **112** 5818–78

[140] Crucho C I C 2024 Silica coatings: from nanostructures to biological entities *Appl. Mater. Today* **38** 102179

[141] Kharisov B I, Dias H V R and Kharissova O V 2019 Mini-review: ferrite nanoparticles in the catalysis *Arab. J. Chem.* **12** 1234–46
[142] Soares P I P, Laia C A T, Carvalho A, Pereira L C J, Coutinho J T, Ferreira I M M, Novo C M M and Borges J P 2016 Iron oxide nanoparticles stabilized with a bilayer of oleic acid for magnetic hyperthermia and MRI applications *Appl. Surf. Sci.* **383** 240–7
[143] Sadjadi S and Sadjadi S 2022 Covalent functionalized silica-coated magnetic nanoparticles: classification, synthetic methods and their applications *Fundamentals and Industrial Applications of Magnetic Nanoparticles* ed C M Hussain and K K Patankar (Cambridge: Woodhead Publishing) ch 4 pp 117–52
[144] Glaria A, Soulé S, Hallali N, Ojo W S, Mirjolet M, Fuks G, Cornejo A, Allouche J, Dupin J C, Martinez H *et al* 2018 Silica coated iron nanoparticles: synthesis, interface control, magnetic and hyperthermia properties *RSC Adv.* **8** 32146–56
[145] Xu Z, Hou Y and Sun S 2007 Magnetic core/shell Fe_3O_4/Au and Fe_3O_4/Au/Ag nanoparticles with tunable plasmonic properties *J. Am. Chem. Soc.* **129** 8698–9
[146] Shahbazi R and Behbahani F K 2024 Synthesis, modifications, and applications of iron-based nanoparticles *Mol. Divers.* **28** 4515–52
[147] Sezer N, Arı İ, Biçer Y and Koç M 2021 Superparamagnetic nanoarchitectures: multimodal functionalities and applications *J. Magn. Magn. Mater.* **538** 168300
[148] Kolhatkar A G, Jamison A C, Litvinov D, Willson R C and Lee T R 2013 Tuning the magnetic properties of nanoparticles *Int. J. Mol. Sci.* **14** 15977–6009
[149] Janjua T I, Cao Y, Kleitz F, Linden M, Yu C and Popat A 2023 Silica nanoparticles: a review of their safety and current strategies to overcome biological barriers *Adv. Drug Deliv. Rev.* **203** 115115
[150] Burlec A F, Corciova A, Boev M, Batir-Marin D, Mircea C, Cioanca O, Danila G, Danila M, Bucur A F and Hancianu M 2023 Current overview of metal nanoparticles' synthesis, characterization, and biomedical applications, with a focus on silver and gold nanoparticles *Pharmaceuticals* **16** 1410
[151] Gao C, Lyu F and Yin Y 2021 Encapsulated metal nanoparticles for catalysis *Chem. Rev.* **121** 834–81
[152] Rodrigues T S, da Silva A G M and Camargo P H C 2019 Nanocatalysis by noble metal nanoparticles: controlled synthesis for the optimization and understanding of activities *J. Mater. Chem.* A **7** 5857–74
[153] Shanker U, Rani M and Hussain C M 2021 *Green Functionalized Nanomaterials for Environmental Applications* (Amsterdam: Elsevier)
[154] Hirsch L R, Gobin A M, Lowery A R, Tam F, Drezek R A, Halas N J and West J L 2006 Metal nanoshells *Ann. Biomed. Eng.* **34** 15–22
[155] Acapulco J A I, Hong S, Kim S K and Park S 2016 Controlling optical properties of metallic multi-shell nanoparticles through suppressed surface plasmon resonance *J. Colloid Interface Sci.* **461** 376–82
[156] Vodyashkin A A, Kezimana P, Prokonov F Y, Vasilenko I A and Stanishevskiy Y M 2022 Current methods for synthesis and potential applications of cobalt nanoparticles: a review *Crystals* **12** 272
[157] Ansari S M, Bhor R D, Pai K R, Sen D, Mazumder S, Ghosh K, Kolekar Y D and Ramana C V 2017 Cobalt nanoparticles for biomedical applications: facile synthesis, physiochemical characterization, cytotoxicity behavior and biocompatibility *Appl. Surf. Sci.* **414** 171–87
[158] Flores-Martinez N, Franceschin G, Gaudisson T, Haj-Khlifa S, Derouich S G, Yaacoub N, Grenèche J-M, Menguy N, Valenzuela R and Ammar S 2019 On the first evidence of

exchange-bias feature in magnetically contrasted consolidates made from $CoFe_2O_4$-CoO core-shell nanoparticles *Sci. Rep.* **9** 19468
[159] Hervault A and Thanh N T K 2014 Magnetic nanoparticle-based therapeutic agents for thermo-chemotherapy treatment of cancer *Nanoscale* **6** 11553–73
[160] Choi W I, Sahu A, Wurm F R and Jo S M 2019 Magnetoliposomes with size controllable insertion of magnetic nanoparticles for efficient targeting of cancer cells *RSC Adv.* **9** 15053–60
[161] Pradhan P, Giri J, Rieken F, Koch C, Mykhaylyk O, Döblinger M, Banerjee R, Bahadur D and Plank C 2010 Targeted temperature sensitive magnetic liposomes for thermo-chemotherapy *J. Control. Release* **142** 108–21
[162] Ta T and Porter T M 2013 Thermosensitive liposomes for localized delivery and triggered release of chemotherapy *J. Control. Release* **169** 112–25
[163] Taléns-Visconti R, Díez-Sales O, de Julián-Ortiz J V and Nácher A 2022 Nanoliposomes in cancer therapy: marketed products and current clinical trials *Int. J. Mol. Sci.* **23** 4249
[164] Nitica S, Fizesan I, Dudric R, Loghin F, Lucaciu C M and Iacovita C 2022 Doxorubicin loaded thermosensitive magneto-liposomes obtained by a gel hydration technique: characterization and *in vitro* magneto-chemotherapeutic effect assessment *Pharmaceutics* **14** 2501
[165] Cepero A, Jiménez-Carretero M, Jabalera Y, Gago L, Luque C, Cabeza L, Melguizo C, Jimenez-Lopez C and Prados J 2024 LGR5 as a therapeutic target of antibody-functionalized biomimetic magnetoliposomes for colon cancer therapy *Int. J. Nanomed.* **19** 1843–65
[166] Miranda M S, Almeida A F, Gomes M E and Rodrigues M T 2022 Magnetic micellar nanovehicles: prospects of multifunctional hybrid systems for precision theranostics *Int. J. Mol. Sci.* **23** 11793
[167] Song Y, Zhu Y, Jiang K, Liu X, Dong L, Li D, Chen S, Xing H, Yan X, Lu Y *et al* 2023 Self-assembling ferrimagnetic fluorescent micelles for bioimaging guided efficient magnetic hyperthermia therapy *Nanoscale* **15** 365–75
[168] Zhang C, Wang X, Liu G, Ren H, Li J, Jiang Z, Liu J, Lovell J F and Zhang Y 2023 Metal coordination micelles for anti-cancer treatment by gene-editing and phototherapy *J. Control. Release* **357** 210–21
[169] Afrouz M, Ahmadi-Nouraldinvand F, Amani A, Zahedian H, Elias S G, Arabnejad F, Yaghoubi H, Farshad O, Farazi N, Jalali A *et al* 2023 Preparation and characterization of magnetic PEG-PEI-PLA-PEI-PEG/Fe_3O_4-PCL/DNA micelles for gene delivery into MCF-7 cells *J. Drug Deliv. Sci. Technol.* **79** 104016
[170] Bhardwaj H and Jangde R K 2023 Current updated review on preparation of polymeric nanoparticles for drug delivery and biomedical applications *Next Nanotechnol.* **2** 100013
[171] Sharifianjazi F, Irani M, Esmaeilkhanian A, Bazli L, Asl M S, Jang H W, Kim S Y, Ramakrishna S, Shokouhimehr M and Varma R S 2021 Polymer incorporated magnetic nanoparticles: applications for magnetoresponsive targeted drug delivery *Mater. Sci. Eng.:* B **272** 115358
[172] Balasubramanian S, Girija A R, Nagaoka Y, Iwai S, Suzuki M, Kizhikkilot V, Yoshida Y, Maekawa T and Nair S D 2014 Curcumin and 5-fluorouracil-loaded, folate- and transferrin-decorated polymeric magnetic nanoformulation: a synergistic cancer therapeutic approach, accelerated by magnetic hyperthermia *Int. J. Nanomed.* **9** 437–59
[173] Senturk F, Cakmak S, Kocum I C, Gumusderelioglu M and Ozturk G G 2021 GRGDS-conjugated and curcumin-loaded magnetic polymeric nanoparticles for the hyperthermia treatment of glioblastoma cells *Colloids Surf.,* A **622** 126648

[174] Mehta P, Sharma M and Devi M 2023 Hydrogels: an overview of its classifications, properties, and applications *J. Mech. Behav. Biomed. Mater.* **147** 106145

[175] Londhe P V, Londhe M V, Salunkhe A B, Laha S S, Mefford O T, Thorat N D and Khot V M 2025 Magnetic hydrogel (MagGel): an evolutionary pedestal for anticancer therapy *Coord. Chem. Rev.* **522** 216228

[176] Derakhshankhah H, Haghshenas B, Eskandani M, Jahanban-Esfahlan R, Abbasi-Maleki S and Jaymand M 2022 Folate-conjugated thermal- and pH-responsive magnetic hydrogel as a drug delivery nano-system for 'smart' chemo/hyperthermia therapy of solid tumors *Mater. Today Commun.* **30** 103148

[177] Eskandani M, Jahanban-Esfahlan R, Sadughi M M and Jaymand M 2024 Thermal-responsive β-cyclodextrin-based magnetic hydrogel as a de novo nanomedicine for chemo/hyperthermia treatment of cancerous cells *Heliyon* **10** e32183

[178] Chavan N, Dharmaraj D, Sarap S and Surve C 2022 Magnetic nanoparticles—a new era in nanotechnology *J. Drug Deliv. Sci. Technol.* **77** 103899

[179] Mukherjee S, Liang L and Veiseh O 2020 Recent advancements of magnetic nanomaterials in cancer therapy *Pharmaceutics* **12** 147

[180] Alonso J, Barandiarán J M, Fernández Barquín L and García-Arribas A 2018 Magnetic nanoparticles, synthesis, properties, and applications *Magnetic Nanostructured Materials* ed A A El-Gendy, J M Barandiarán and R L Hadimani (Amsterdam: Elsevier) ch 1 pp 1–40

[181] Duan M, Shapter J G, Qi W, Yang S and Gao G 2018 Recent progress in magnetic nanoparticles: synthesis, properties, and applications *Nanotechnology* **29** 452001

[182] Estelrich J, Escribano E, Queralt J and Busquets M A 2015 Iron oxide nanoparticles for magnetically-guided and magnetically-responsive drug delivery *Int. J. Mol. Sci.* **16** 8070–101

[183] Chorny M, Hood E, Levy R J and Muzykantov V R 2010 Endothelial delivery of antioxidant enzymes loaded into non-polymeric magnetic nanoparticles *J. Control. Release* **146** 144–51

[184] Amatya R, Hwang S, Park T, Min K A and Shin M C 2021 In vitro and *in vivo* evaluation of PEGylated starch-coated iron oxide nanoparticles for enhanced photothermal cancer therapy *Pharmaceutics* **13** 871

[185] García-García G, Lázaro M, Cenalmor A, García-Álvarez I, Iglesias G R and Arias J L 2024 Cluster/shell citrate-Fe_3O_4/chitosan nanoparticles for enhancing heating efficiency in combined magnetic and photothermal therapy *Ceram. Int.* **50** 36295–305

[186] Ying Y, Zhou Y, Yu J, Qiao L, Zheng J, Li W, Li J and Che S 2024 Preparation of dextran- and carboxymethyl dextran–coated Fe_3O_4 nanoparticles for breast cancer cell labeling and magnetic hyperthermia *J. Supercond. Nov. Magn.* **37** 1453–63

[187] Iqbal Y, Hussain Shah W, Yaqoob Khan M, Ahmed P, Tauseef Qureshi M, Mohamed Khaled A and Syed Salem M 2024 Optimizing the magnetic field strength and concentration of silica coated cobalt ferrite nanoparticles for magnetic hyperthermia *Inorg. Chem. Commun.* **167** 112796

[188] Shava B, Ayodeji F D, Rahdar A, Iqbal H M N and Bilal M 2022 Magnetic nanoparticles-based systems for multifaceted biomedical applications *J. Drug Deliv. Sci. Technol.* **74** 103616

[189] Flores-Rojas G G, López-Saucedo F, Vera-Graziano R, Mendizabal E and Bucio E 2022 Magnetic nanoparticles for medical applications: updated review *Macromol* **2** 374–90

Sudip Mukherjee, Vijay Sagar Madamsetty, Lipi Pradhan, Anjali Upadhyay and Devyani Yenurkar

Chapter 2

Synthesis of MNPs and their physicochemical characterization

Magnetic nanoparticles (MNPs), for example, silver, cobalt, iron, and gold, have attracted much attention due to their many applications in various disciplines and low toxicity to people. MNPs can be synthesized using various physical, chemical, and biological methods. These techniques offer significant control over the size and size distribution of the MNPs. X-ray diffraction (XRD), scanning electron microscopy (SEM), transmission electron microscopy (TEM), Fourier transform infrared (FTIR) spectroscopy, and inductively coupled plasma mass spectrometry (ICPMS) have been used to characterize MNPs. The primary synthetic techniques for MNPs, along with their characterizations, are briefly covered in this chapter. We then discuss the potential applications of MNPs in different biological systems.

In recent years, nanoparticles (NPs) have gained popularity in a variety of industrial applications due to their remarkable properties [1]. Out of these NPs, MNPs have garnered much interest because of their unique nanoscale characteristics, namely their magnetic activity [2, 3]. MNPs are a unique type of NP that has superparamagnetic, ferrimagnetic, and ferromagnetic characteristics; they can interact with an external magnetic field. Materials that have nanoscale dimensions, usually ranging from 1 to 100 nanometers, are called MNPs [4]. They differ from their bulk counterparts at this scale due to peculiar magnetic characteristics that appear. According to a healthcare report, the market for MNPs was calculated to have reached USD 48.4 million in 2022 and is projected to increase at a substantial compound annual growth rate (CAGR) of 10.3% from 2023 to 2028 to reach USD 96.2 million. Typically, MNPs are made up of atoms, ions, or molecules with a net nonzero magnetic dipole moment that primarily comes from the presence of unpaired electrons. Examples include iron, cobalt, nickel, Gd, and their alloys with AuFe, NiCo, $Nd_2Fe_{14}B$, and SmCo; and their oxides or carbides, such as Fe_2O_3, Fe_3O_4, NiO, CoO, Gd_2O_3, $Gd_3Fe_5O_{12}$, MnO, Mn_3O_4, $Zn_{1-x}Mn_xO$, $CoFe_2O_4$, Cr_2O_3, Fe_3C, and Co_3C, among others. When an ensemble's MNPs are made up of various kinds of

doi:10.1088/978-0-7503-6335-8ch2 © IOP Publishing Ltd 2025. All rights, including for text and data mining (TDM), artificial intelligence (AI) training, and similar technologies, are reserved.

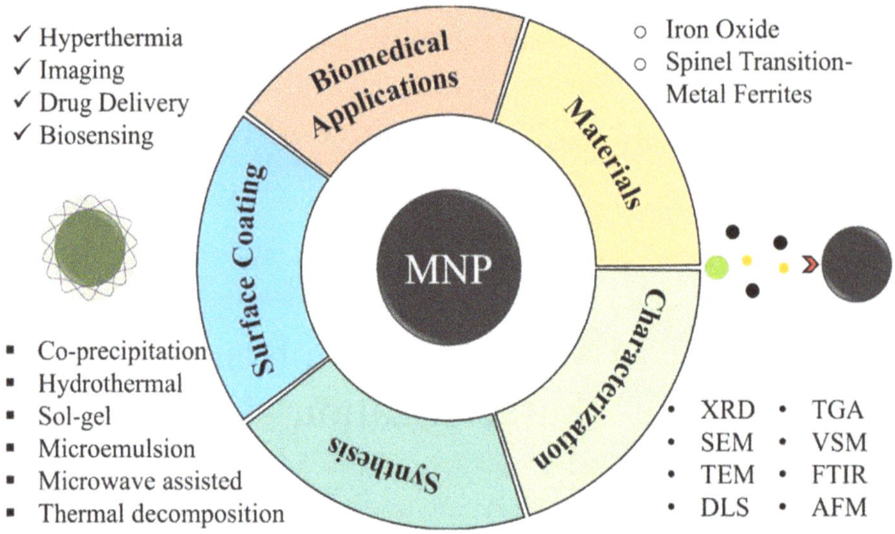

Figure 2.1. Overview of the topics covered in this chapter [15] John Wiley & Sons. © 2023 Wiley-VCH GmbH.

magnetic materials, the characteristics of every kind of magnetic material are superimposed to determine the ensemble's magnetic characteristics [5].

Several techniques are used in their synthesis to regulate the dimensions, characteristics, and form of these nanoscale materials. Chemical techniques are frequently employed, particularly sol–gel synthesis, coprecipitation, and thermal decomposition [6]. Furthermore, biological techniques, such as biomimetic synthesis employing microbes or plant extracts, provide environmentally favorable substitutes [7]. On the other hand, physical techniques provide fine control over the size of NPs but may call for specialized tools and regulated settings [8].

MNPs are commonly used in the theranostic field because of their multifunctional properties. They are used in drug delivery [9], radiology, cell labeling, magnetic cell sorting schemes [10], and in making nanobiosensors [11]. MNPs are also used in magnetic resonance imaging (MRI) as contrast-enhancing agents [12]. The application of MNPs in cancer therapy, targeted medication, gene delivery, intra- and extracellular hyperthermia (HT), and cancer theranostics is now the focus of much research [13, 14]. The use of these MNPs in the various fields of biology mostly depends on their physical and chemical properties, such as size, composition, biocompatibility, and toxicity.

In this chapter, we present the various methods of MNP synthesis, the characterization of MNPs, their physical and chemical properties, and how these properties can be used for biological applications such as therapeutics, diagnosis, etc (figure 2.1) [15].

2.1 Various methods for MNP synthesis

Various physical, chemical, and biological techniques are used to create MNPs, as shown in figure 2.2. Selecting the proper synthesis technique aids in creating MNPs with the required size, shape, structure, colloidal stability, and magnetic

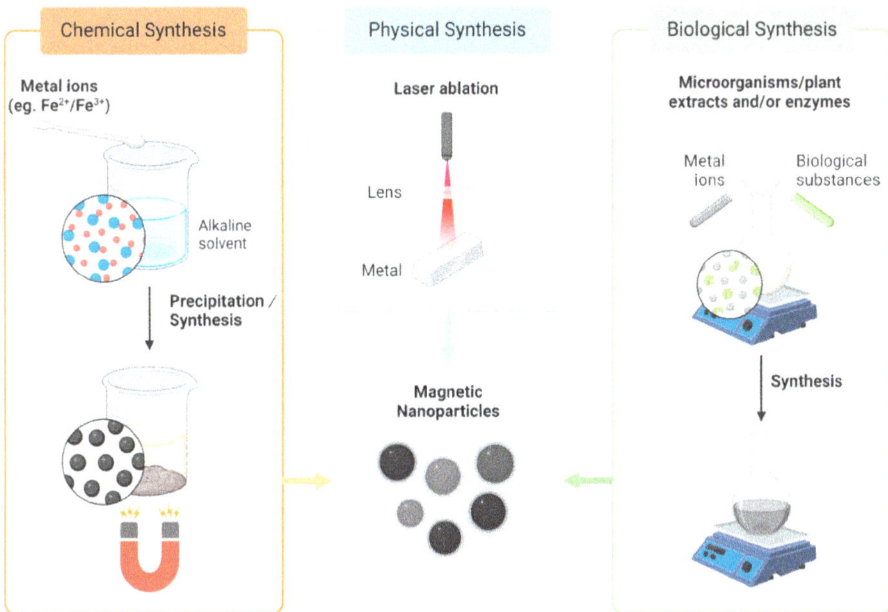

Figure 2.2. Different methods for MNP synthesis. Adapted from [17]. CC BY 4.0.

characteristics. These characteristics of MNPs are crucial in determining their range of use. The most popular strategy among the techniques listed above is chemical coprecipitation [16].

2.1.1 Physical synthesis methods

Different physical techniques can be used to create MNPs, and each has unique benefits in terms of homogeneity, size control, and functional characteristics. Some of the physical methods used for MNP synthesis and their advantages are listed below.

2.1.1.1 Gas-phase deposition

The production of MNPs through gas-phase deposition is a sophisticated method that allows precise control over the NPs' size, shape, and composition. The two main gas-phase deposition techniques are physical vapor deposition (PVD) and chemical vapor deposition (CVD). PVD can generate composite NPs and thin films by either thermally treating composites on a surface within an inert environment or through the supersaturation of precursor molecules in the gas phase. This process results in fine MNPs, nanocomposites, thin films, and fine particulate powders [18–21]. On the other hand, CVD is commonly used for producing high-quality iron oxide nanotubes or thin films. A key advantage of gas-phase deposition over liquid-based synthesis is the greater purity of the resulting particles, as the absence of water prevents the introduction of microorganisms and other impurities [8]. An example of this method is the work by Hammad *et al* who synthesized iron oxide NPs using a gas-phase technique and applied them to enhance HT treatment [22].

2.1.1.2 Electron-beam lithography

By focusing an electron beam onto a substrate covered in a thin layer of resin, electron beam lithography can remove only the exposed or unexposed portions of the resin [23]. This technique allows for the synthesis of NPs, producing smaller and more precise particles than traditional methods such as photolithography [24]. It has been extensively utilized to fabricate nanorods with magnetic properties and nanorings with thin films of metal oxides that are spin-coated with an organic resin [25]. During the process, the metal oxide film is immersed in a bath containing a solvent, and a tightly focused beam of electrons is used to make patterns on it. This process removes and evaporates the excess metal, causing NPs smaller than 50 nm to develop [26].

2.1.1.3 Laser-induced pyrolysis

Large-scale production via laser pyrolysis involves varying a gaseous precursor's vapor pressure and adjusting the fuel and air ratio during the heating process. Pyrolysis is frequently used to make particles with an average size of 2–7 nm [27]. A continuous-wave CO_2 laser is used in the laser pyrolysis process to heat a flowing mixture of gases, starting and maintaining a chemical reaction. Gavrila-Florescu *et al* used the laser-induced pyrolysis process in an oxygen-deficient atmosphere to create nanosized iron-based core ZnO shell particles in a single step. They explored the anticancer efficacy of the synthesized particles and also examined the cytotoxic effect of the NPs on normal cells [28]. Kongkaew *et al* used laser ablation to synthesize gold NP–polypyrrole–chitosan on graphene for ascorbic acid detection [29].

2.1.1.4 High-energy ball milling

This method creates fine, homogeneous oxide NPs with good dispersion by subjecting the powdered mixture to high-energy collisions in a mill in the presence of balls. The powdered mixes must be balanced throughout the ball milling process to create cold-welded and fractured alloys [30]. The rotation time and speed greatly influence the size and characteristics of iron oxide NPs. This process can use various mill types, including the planetary method, oscillation of the material and the mill, and vibrating mills. The planetary mill is considered the most efficient for producing iron oxide NPs because a container of millings can rotate on two parallel axes, mimicking a planet's orbit around the sun, enhancing the milling efficiency and particle refinement [31]. Chen *et al* utilized the simple ball milling method to synthesize dextran-coated supermagnetic iron oxide NPs [32]. Velásquez *et al* demonstrated that mechanical milling in the presence of polyethylene glycol (PEG) is a straightforward and efficient method for producing magnetite–maghemite NPs with favorable mechanical properties, making them suitable for applications in nanotechnology [33]. Wirunchit *et al*'s synthesis of ZnO NPs by ball milling is shown in figure 2.3.

2.1.1.5 Hydrothermal and solvothermal methods

According to published literature, the hydrothermal and solvothermal methods are preparation methods used to synthesize MNPs and ultrafine powders. One option is

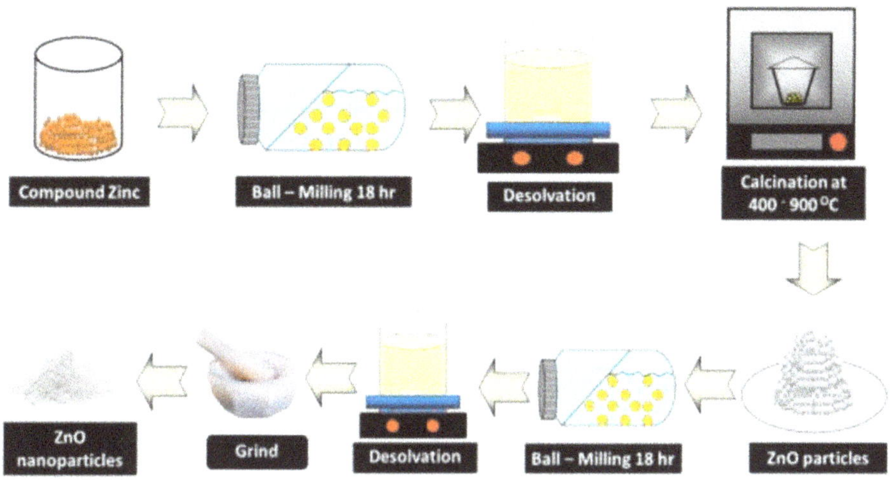

Figure 2.3. Synthesis of Zn oxide NPs by the ball milling method. Adapted from [34], Copyright (2021), with permission from Elsevier.

the hydrothermal process, which uses various wet chemical methods to crystallize NPs from solution in a sealed hydrothermal container at very high temperatures (between 130 °C and 250 °C) and vapor pressures (typically between 0.3 and 4 MPa) [35]. In hydrothermal processes, precursor materials are dissolved in a solvent, usually water, and the solution is then heated to high pressure and temperature inside a sealed reactor. Through nucleation and subsequent particle growth, this environment promotes the development of NPs [36]. Kurian *et al* synthesized a highly efficient magnetic fluid for HT using copper ferrite ($CuFe_2O_4$) NPs. Because of its PEG coating, *in vitro* cytotoxicity experiments showed that the copper ferrite–PEG (CF–PEG) MNPs were biocompatible with human colon epithelial cells (HT-29). The solvothermally produced $CuFe_2O_4$ MNPs were suitable for magnetic fluid HT, as evidenced by their excellent heating efficiency, negligible room temperature coercivity, and superior biocompatibility [37]. Fotukian *et al* used the solvothermal synthesis method to synthesize $CuFe_2O_4$ and Fe_3O_4 NPs, which exhibited heating efficacy in magnetic HT (MHT) applications. The particle size of the NPs was also maintained up to 50 nm, which is essential for their use in HT [38]. Pathak *et al* synthesized iron oxide NPs using the hydrothermal method, as shown in figure 2.4 [39].

2.1.2 Chemical synthesis methods

2.1.2.1 Coprecipitation method

Coprecipitation is the most popular and appropriate technique for creating MNPs with controlled sizes and magnetic properties. This process creates MNPs from aqueous salt solutions by mixing them with a base at ambient or high temperatures in an inert environment. This method is generally used to synthesize metal oxides and ferrites [40]. Numerous studies have established different synthesis strategies,

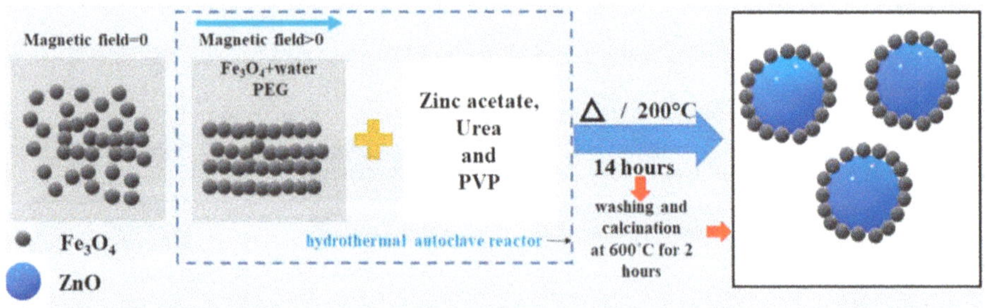

Figure 2.4. Diagram showing the altered hydrothermal method used to create the Fe_3O_4 surface-adorned ZnO nanocomposite. Adapted from [39]. CC BY 4.0.

with the chemical coprecipitation method emerging as a highly effective method for generating stable, homogeneous, and finely crystalline NPs [16, 41]. Houshiar *et al* synthesized cobalt ferrite ($CoFe_2O_4$) using the pyrolytic and coprecipitation methods and compared the size, structure, and magnetic properties of the resulting materials. They found that the different synthesis methods resulted in different particle sizes and magnetic properties. The magnetic properties of the NPs synthesized by the pyrolytic method were stronger than those of the NPs synthesized using the coprecipitation method [42]. Petcharoen *et al* synthesized MNPs via the coprecipitation method and characterized them. Every magnetite NP exhibited significant saturation magnetization and superparamagnetic behavior. Additionally, magnetite NPs coated with hexanoic acid had the maximum magnetization, measuring 58.72 emu g^{-1} [43]. Babu *et al* [44] studied the characteristics of catalysts based on copper tin hydroxide made using the coprecipitation method for the photocatalytic degradation of methylene blue dye.

2.1.2.2 Thermal decomposition

Thermal decomposition is also known as thermolysis. This refers to the method of breaking down a material by applying heat. The heat at which a chemical undergoes decomposition is called its thermal decomposition temperature. Since this procedure requires heat to break chemical bonds, it is classified as an endothermic reaction. Various types of MNPs, including Mn, Co, and Zn MNPs, have been synthesized using this technique [45]. This method is particularly effective in producing iron oxide MNPs with useful properties, typically with a particle size of 15 nm [46]. By utilizing organic solubilizing agents and surfactants like fatty acids and oleic acid, the high-temperature degradation of organometallic substrates, such as [Mn^+(acac)*n*] (where M represents iron, manganese, cobalt, nickel, or chromium, $n = 2$ or 3, and acac = acetylacetonate) or carbonyls like $Fe(CO)_5$, allows for precise control over NP size and uniformity [40]. Hyeon *et al* successfully synthesized monodisperse γ-Fe_2O_3 NPs by thermally decomposing iron pentacarbonyl and oleic acid at 100 °C, followed by oxidizing the by-product iron–oleic acid complex to produce maghemite (γ-Fe_2O_3) particles [47]. Moreover, Sánchez *et al* synthesized $Mn_xGa_{1-x}Fe_2O_4$ MNPs through thermal decomposition for medical diagnostic applications. Numerous studies have explored the synthesis of MNPs using this process for various biomedical applications [48, 49].

2.1.2.3 Sol–gel method

The sol–gel process is commonly used for the synthesis of various iron oxide MNPs and silica-tagged MNPs. Large numbers of MNPs with a controlled size and distinct shape can be manufactured using this method [50]. MNPs were previously made by heating a solution of $FeCl_3$ and NaOH to between 50 °C and 100 °C. The sol–gel method is a less expensive technology because it does not require any specific equipment and can be carried out at ambient temperature. This technology can easily control the composition, size, and form of MNPs. This process yields extremely pure solid materials with good crystallinity and tunability. However, this process occasionally produces contamination due to byproduct reactions, necessitating retreatment to obtain pure MNPs [51]. The creation of three-dimensional oxide networks limits its effectiveness in producing dispersed NPs. Other drawbacks include this method's use of hazardous organic solvents and lengthy reaction times. Moradnia *et al* synthesized magnetic $Mg_{0.5}Zn_{0.5}FeMnO_4$ NPs by the sol–gel method for a photocatalytic application [52]. Esmaeilkhanian *et al* evaluated the cytotoxicity of thermoresponsive core/shell $Ni_xCo_{1-x}Fe_2O_4$/PEG NPs synthesized by the sol–gel method [53]. Endla *et al* demonstrated the use of the sol–gel method to synthesize cobalt-doped MgO NPs, as presented in [51].

2.1.2.4 Microwave-assisted synthesis

Because microwave technology can heat precursor components quickly and uniformly, it has been used to synthesize MNPs. Microwave irradiation's penetrating ability enables homogeneous heating of the reaction solution, which promotes uniform crystallization and the quick development of crystallites with a limited size distribution. Microwaves' electric and magnetic components work together to create friction and molecular collisions, which speed up reaction times compared to traditional techniques. Consequently, uniformly sized and shaped MNPs appropriate for biomedical applications, especially functional imaging, can be produced by microwave-assisted synthesis [54]. Brollo *et al*'s work indicates that microwave-assisted synthesis is essential for creating exceptional MNPs. The experimental conditions, including the solvent, precursor, and surfactant, ultimately determine particle size and homogeneity. These parameters have a significant impact on the nucleation and growth processes. In contrast to traditional heating techniques, microwave heating offers efficient internal heating that encourages nucleation across the reaction solution and restricts the possibility of numerous nuclei developing. According to research, this method can produce MNPs with diameters between 8 and 15 nm. These particles, which are suitable candidates for use as MRI negative contrast agents, exhibit superparamagnetic behavior when synthesized through microwave and thermal decomposition in organic environments. The main parameters influencing these NPs' efficacy as MRI contrast agents seem to be their tiny hydrodynamic diameters and saturation magnetization (M_s) [55].

2.1.3 Biological synthesis

Biological approaches appear to be a good substitute for physical and chemical methods, since they offer safer, more environmentally friendly, and less energy-intensive synthesis [56]. The disadvantages of the previously listed techniques (such as high costs, the use of toxic and hazardous chemicals, and the creation of hazardous reaction byproducts) are avoided by biological synthesis, which presupposes the combination of metal atoms from metal precursors with NPs in green substrates [57, 58]. Two major groups can be distinguished based on the biological substrate: synthesis methods based on plants and those based on microorganisms, especially bacteria [59].

Research into the bacteria-mediated synthesis technique suggests that magnetotactic and iron-reducing bacteria can produce single-domain MNPs in extracellular or intracellular anaerobic environments [59]. The primary benefits of employing bacteria as reactors are their quick growth and simplicity in cultivation and modification [60]. Compared to other traditional techniques, bacterial fermentation produces high-quality products with fewer faults or dislocations and is scalable and reproducible [61]. However, magnetotactic bacteria must grow quickly, which is challenging to achieve in artificial laboratory settings, making the process time-consuming and costly [62]. Elblbesy *et al* synthesized magnetite NPs using the *Magnetospirillum* strain AMB-1. They synthesized NPs with a size of 47 nm and investigated their magnetic properties, such as hysteresis loop, saturation magnetization, and coercivity, which were measured at different temperatures [63]. However, plant-based synthesis is thought to be the most effective way to create NPs quickly. Different substrates, including callus, leaf, fruit, and seed extracts, can be used in plant-based techniques to create particles with saturation magnetization and mean sizes appropriate for biological applications [58]. Iron oxide NPs smaller than 50 nm were created by Buonu *et al* utilizing *Psidium guajava* and *Moringa oleifera* extracts. Based on their findings, they claimed that these iron oxide NPs have the ability to degrade bacteria and methylene blue through photocatalysis [64]. *Moringa oleifera* leaf extract was utilized to synthesize iron oxide MNPs with a rod-like shape. These nanorods exhibited superparamagnetism and had an average NP size of 15 nm. Rod-shaped iron oxide MNPs were reported to have very good antibacterial activity, similar to that of spherical iron oxide NPs [65]. Extracts from *Azadirachta indica* have been utilized to initiate the production of iron oxide NPs [66]. Various methods of synthesis of MNPs are summarized in table 2.1.

2.2 Physicochemical characterization of MNPs

MNPs are mostly characterized by using various instrumentation to analyze their physicochemical characteristics, which are crucial for determining the probable effectiveness of MNPs for their delivery target. To successfully reach their target, MNPs must overcome two primary challenges: physiological barriers and cellular barriers [78, 79]. The diverse structural, physical, chemical, magnetic, and electrical properties of MNPs enable a broad spectrum of applications, enhancing their potential. MNPs offer numerous benefits, such as ease of separation, regeneration, and reusability, which help reduce operating costs [80]. The size, shape, and composition of MNPs also influence their magnetic characteristics, making precise characterization essential for determining the reproducibility of the results [81]. For

Table 2.1. Various methods used to synthesize MNPs, with their advantages and disadvantages.

S. No.	Synthesis method	Advantages	Disadvantages	References
1.	Gas-phase deposition	• Scalability. • Cost-effective • Size and composition control. • Shape and size control	• Hazardous reactants • Low yield • Agglomeration	[67, 68]
2.	Sol–gel	• High purity • Uniformity • Rapid synthesis • Versatile	• Complex synthesis process. • Safety issue • Low scalability • Maximum time for synthesis • High cost	[69]
3.	Electron-beam lithography	• High resolution • Good reliability and accuracy	• Very expensive and complex • Slower than many such techniques	[60]
4.	Power ball milling	• Versatile • Simple and economical • Adjustable reaction conditions	• Wear of grinding media • Excessive heat and residual strain	[70]
5.	Coprecipitation	• Narrow size distribution • Strong magnetic properties • High purity	• Particle aggregation • Risk of contamination • Limited compositional control	[71]
6.	Microemulsion	• Control of size and shape • Narrow size distribution	• Complex formulation • Potential contamination • Limited morphological control	[72]
7.	Polyol	• High stability • Low cost • Controlled size and shape • High purity	• Limited morphological control • Potential toxicity • Limited material selection	[73]

(Continued)

Table 2.1. (*Continued*)

S. No.	Synthesis method	Advantages	Disadvantages	References
8.	Microwave	• Low cost • Scalability • Controlled size and shape • Uniformity	• Limited reproducibility • Limited control of surface chemistry • Safety concerns	[74]
9.	Solvothermal	• Wide selection of materials • Tailored surface properties • Control of size and shape	• High production cost • Lengthy procedure • Limited scalability	[75]
10.	Sonochemical	• Versatility • Low cost	• Limited scalability • Low uniformity • Little control over surface chemistry	[76]
11.	Biological	• Biocompatibility • Environmental sustainability • Cost-effective and high yield	• Difficulty controlling size and shape • Weak NP dispersion • Attachment of active molecules	[77]

instance, while variation in MNP structure promotes inhomogeneity, a decrease in their size results in unexceptional magnetism. Furthermore, identifying the most effective synthesis strategy that may improve the MNPs' target-specific capacity depends on the validity and dependability of several characterization techniques [82]. The tools commonly used for characterizing MNPs include SEM, energy-dispersive x-ray diffraction (EDXD), atomic force microscopy (AFM), TEM, Mössbauer spectroscopy (MS), UV spectrophotometry, and FTIR spectroscopy [83]. Some important physiochemical properties of MNPs and their characterization techniques are given below.

2.2.1 Size, shape, and surface morphology

Physicochemical properties, such as the size and shape of MNPs, play an important role in their stability. The particle size greatly influences the magnetic moment and responsiveness. The dynamic light scattering (DLS) and Brunauer–Emmett–Teller (BET) methods are used to measure surface area, size, and particle dispersion. However, methods such as AFM, TEM/high-resolution TEM (HRTEM), and

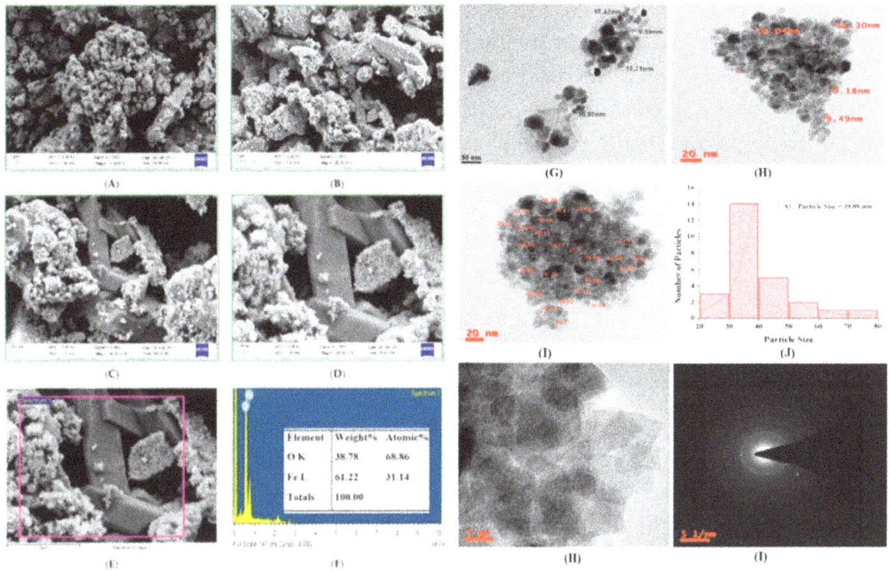

Figure 2.5. Characterization of iron oxide NPs: (A–D) SEM images, (E) electron diffraction spectroscopy (EDS) spot, (F) EDS spectrum, (G–I) TEM images, (H) histogram, (I) D-spacing and lattice fringes, and (J) selected area electron diffraction (SAED) pattern. Adapted from [88]. CC BY 4.0.

SEM/field emission SEM (FESEM) can identify MNPs' surface shape. We may determine their diameter by using the images we obtain from these instruments, which give us a sense of their size and shape. The position of scattered particles, step height, and surface roughness are all measured using the AFM technique. TEM provides information about the size, shape, and composition of NPs. SEM offers valuable information about the composition and surface topography of samples. When the nanomaterials' surface is nonconductive, ultrathin electrically conducting elements are applied through sputtering. Particle size can be determined using techniques such as XRD, FESEM, and HRTEM. TEM is particularly useful for assessing crystallinity, NP aggregation, lattice spacing, and electron phase shift [84–86]. The Scherrer equation provides a straightforward method for determining NP size from the sharp peaks in XRD patterns. However, noncrystalline MNPs exhibit wide peaks, making size determination more difficult. XRD is used to assess the crystallinity of NPs. A study by Reddy *et al* suggested that reduced NP size, which maximizes surface area, may affect the noncrystalline properties of MNPs and, consequently, their magnetic moments [87]. Virendra *et al* synthesized iron oxide MNPs for wastewater treatment. They performed various characterizations, such as SEM, DLS, and TEM, to analyze the shape, morphology, and size of the NPs, as shown in figure 2.5(A–I).

2.2.2 Elemental mapping/composition

Surface morphology and elemental components of NPs can be determined using various instruments, such as electron diffraction spectroscopy (EDS)/EDXD, x-ray fluorescence (XRF), TEM, SEM, and x-ray photoelectron spectroscopy (XPS). Additionally, the elemental composition can be analyzed using atomic absorption spectrophotometry (AAS) and ICPMS. However, AAS cannot directly determine the elemental makeup of solid NPs, as they must first be dissolved in acids or bases. XPS effectively identifies the chemical state and content of elements within the NPs. The EDXD method is also valuable for elemental analysis and determining the chemical composition of MNPs [40]. XRF can provide information on a sample's elemental composition. Compared to alternative techniques, XRF analysis sample preparation is simple, quick, and secure. It can detect elements at up to 100 parts per billion, or ppb [89, 90].

2.2.3 Bonding type and structure

Several methods are used to ascertain the structure and bonding properties of MNPs. The methods include FTIR spectroscopy, Raman spectroscopy (RS), thermogravimetric analysis (TGA), x-ray absorption spectroscopy (XAS), and XPS. The surface configuration of NPs can be examined using XPS, which also offers information on the structural properties and speciation of elements and exposes the reaction mechanisms occurring on MNP particle surfaces [91]. FTIR and XPS are useful tools for determining the oxidation state, particle binding energy, and organic–inorganic bonding. Another benefit of using FTIR spectroscopy is obtaining an understanding of the functional groups of organic compounds. The compound's structure and crystal lattice are determined using the RS method. The TGA approach gives us information regarding the formation of coatings, particularly surfactants and polymers, and is utilized to assess binding efficacy on particle surfaces. Information on oxidation states and necessary components of the electronic configuration can be found using the XAS approach [87].

2.2.4 Magnetism

Determining NPs' magnetic properties is important for assessing their stability, effectiveness, recovery, and recyclability [92]. When taken out of a magnetic field, paramagnetic particles do not exhibit any lasting magnetic property, but ferromagnetic NPs exhibit permanent magnetization over time [82]. Magnetic induction (B) and magnetic field strength (H) are the main determinants of NPs' magnetism or magnetic characteristics. B and H generally have a linear relationship controlled by the magnetic permeability (μ) of NPs. If μ is greater than one, the MNPs are paramagnetic; if μ is less than one, they are diamagnetic [87]. Because of this magnetic characteristic, MNPs may be essential for regulated therapy and focused drug delivery. Several methods are used to test the magnetism of NPs, and they differ in sensitivity and information quality. Total magnetization is measured using superconducting quantum interference device (SQUID) magnetometry and vibrating sample magnetometry (VSM). SQUID is particularly useful for analyzing samples in various states, including thin film surfaces, crystals, powders, liquids, and gases. SQUID and VSM are extremely sensitive; for example, SQUID magnetometry can detect as little as 10^{-10} emu, while VSM can detect as little as 10^{-6} emu [39, 93]. Another trustworthy method for measuring the magnetic characteristics and behavior of NPs is the physical property measurement system (PPMS). This apparatus is used to detect the temperature and magnetization of MNP samples within a magnetic field [93].

2.3 Thermodynamic influences on MNP self-assembly and therapeutic uses

Understanding the forces influencing MNPs' self-assembly requires an understanding of their thermodynamics. MNPs may scatter or form stable structures, depending on the balance between stabilizing and destabilizing forces. An outline of these forces and their thermodynamic functions is given here. In thermodynamics, self-assembly arranges structural units into larger structures, including atoms, molecules, or NPs. These structures can take on intricate shapes and are stabilized against thermal disruption by the system's inherent nanoscale forces of interaction [94]. The use of a nanostructured containing surface (template) or external fields can initiate the self-assembly process [95, 96]. In this context, the field guides the self-assembly process and determines the final structures that form, including their defect density, dimensionality, and anisotropy. In nanomagnetic systems, the primary mechanism driving self-assembly is the magnetostatic dipole–dipole interaction, which is the dominant factor in the interactions between MNPs. The energy required to move two NPs with magnetic dipole moments m_1 and m_2 from an infinite distance to a finite separation is called the dipole–dipole interaction energy [97, 98]. Directionality is crucial for magnetic dipole–dipole interactions. Two patterns in the self-assembly process emerge when an external magnetic field is applied: first, even for extremely small particles that would not typically aggregate readily in the absence of the field, the external magnetic field may cause the development of NP arrays [99, 100]; second, oriented anisotropic structures are created, such as string phases that are oriented in relation to the field. Even the possibility of a reversible field-assisted self-assembly process has been demonstrated. For MNPs, various other interactions must be considered in addition to magnetic ones. These could include the repulsive forces from the surfactant chains and the van der Waals attraction between metallic cores. As particle size decreases, van der Waals forces become more significant. This conclusion can be reached even by considering spherical particles covered with a self-assembled monolayer (SAM). The magnetic cores are kept at least $\sim$2 d apart by the surface defect layer, preventing them from coming into contact [98, 101]. The Derjaguin approximation states that ($d \ll a$) holds true when d is more or less than the NP diameter. For instance, as mentioned, the van der Waals interaction between particles primarily occurs in 10 nm γ-Fe_2O_3 NPs when no external magnetic field is present. In contrast, the self-assembly of this system is dominated and governed by magnetic interactions when there is a strong external magnetic field [99]. Various destabilizing forces also influence MNP assembly.

2.4 Use of MNPs in therapeutic applications

MNPs have gained significant popularity due to their promising results across various fields. Their superparamagnetic characteristics, specific size and shape, high surface area-to-volume ratio, and biocompatibility make them appealing. In this section, we provide a detailed analysis of the applications of MNPs in several well-known areas. Because of their physicochemical characteristics, ease of manufacture, stability, and biocompatibility, MNPs have recently found extensive use in various biological applications. When exposed to external magnetic forces, MNPs can interact with them. By changing nearby magnetic fields, MNPs can improve MRI as well as cancer therapeutics. Depending on their specific application, MNPs made from different materials display varying physical and magnetic properties. However, the most crucial element in biomedical research is their potential toxicity or biocompatibility [102, 103].

2.4.1 In cancer treatment

In recent decades, molecular biology and nanobiotechnological sciences have become innovative approaches to cancer theranostics [104, 105]. This has mainly taken place through the development of advanced NPs with maximized properties to address the drawbacks of previous cancer treatment and diagnostic methods, as shown in figure 2.6 [106, 107]. Through improved infiltration and retention, NPs are also being developed as vehicles to efficiently transfer genes, proteins, or anticancer medicines to targeted tumor locations [108].

Despite the promise of existing NPs, new NPs that can fulfill the demands of developing cancer theranostics are desperately needed. In this regard, MNPs are excellent candidates for the detection and treatment of cancer because of their special physicochemical qualities and superparamagnetic traits. MNPs are very reactive; they have a huge surface-area-to-mass ratio and a diameter of about 100 nm [109].

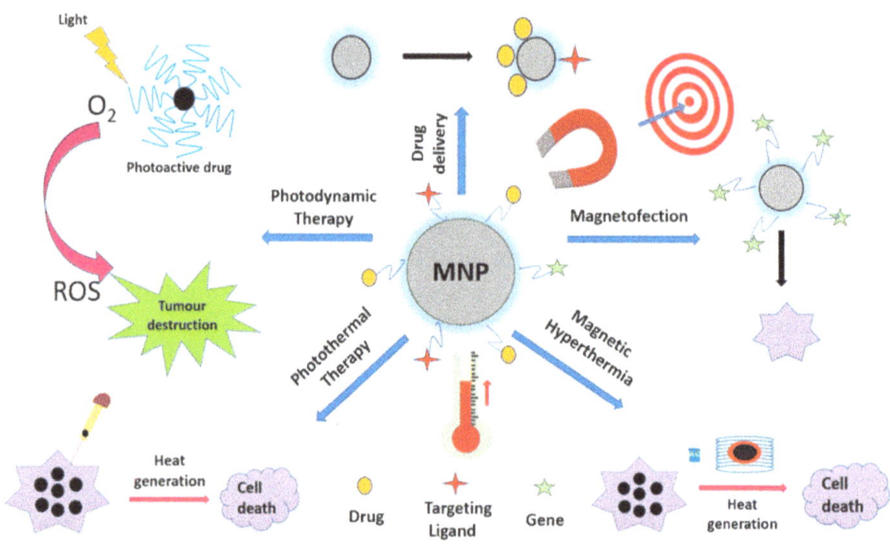

Figure 2.6. Applications of MNPs in cancer therapy. Adapted from [110] with permission from the Royal Society of Chemistry.

2.4.1.1 Use of MNPs for cancer treatment by magnetic hyperthermia

Treatment for HT involves the application of increased heat over a localized tissue area, causing irreversibly pathogenic targets to be heated to a high temperature. An external alternating magnetic field (AMF) is used to create heat in MNP suspensions inside the body in a novel cancer treatment called MHT (figure 2.7) [109, 111]. MNPs can localize heat produced by an AMF for non-invasive HT. Iron oxide NPs are the most promising thermosensitizers for application in HT because of their size, ease of functionalization with both organic and inorganic chemicals, biocompatibility, minimal toxicity, and ease of excretion [112]. Furthermore, MNPs' ferromagnetic characteristics can be used for both diagnostic and therapeutic purposes. Theranostic activity is a characteristic of iron oxide NPs. MNPs are crucial components of diagnostic systems that track disease progression and the efficacy of treatment. Furthermore, MNPs are employed as parts of intricate drug delivery systems for nucleic acids, immunomodulators, and anticancer medications [113]. When MNPs are subjected to an electromagnetic field, their oscillatory vibrations cause a localized rise in temperature and a release of cargo, such as anticancer medications [114, 115]. Using a mouse xenograft model, Zhao *et al* described the use of MNPs to treat head and neck malignancies. According to the results, the tumor center's temperature rose sharply from body temperature to 40 °C in 5–10 min. The treated tumor tissue developed necrosis as a result of this hyperthermic treatment [116]. Hu *et al* similarly treated mouse lung cancer models with MHT. The results demonstrated that apoptosis was induced, decreasing tumor development [117]. The effectiveness of oleic-acid-coated SIONPs for MHT of murine fibrosarcoma tumor models was recently shown by Shetake *et al.* The results indicated that MHT significantly reduced tumor growth by altering the heat shock protein 90 (HSP 90)/AKT pathway to induce apoptosis [118]. Additionally, a case study has

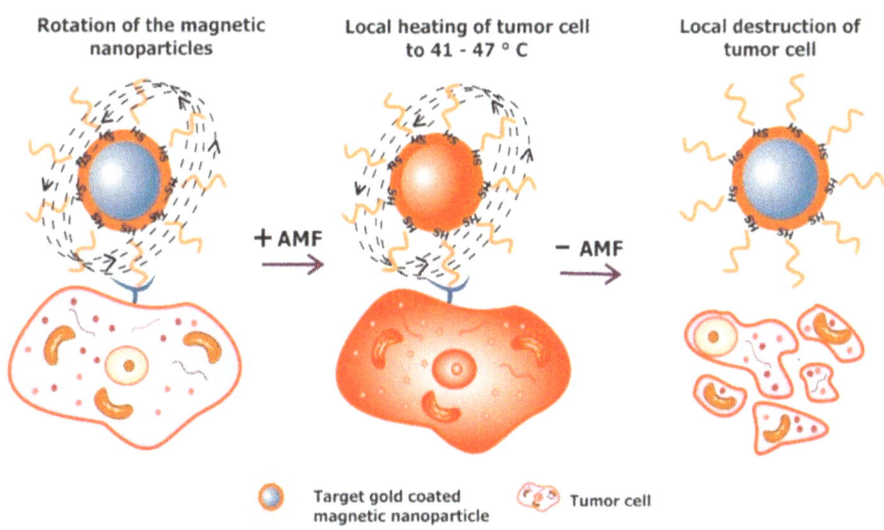

Figure 2.7. HT treatment of cancer using MNPs. Adapted with permission from [120]. CC BY 4.0.

demonstrated the effectiveness of MHT in conjunction with chemotherapy (gemcitabine/cisplatin) for a patient having a cholangiocarcinoma removed. A 54-year-old man was given preoperative chemoradiation and neoadjuvant therapy after being diagnosed with hilar cholangiocarcinoma (also known as a Klatskin tumor). However, he chose to undergo chemotherapy and HT as a result of the unsuccessful radiation and chemotherapy treatments. After 32 rounds of chemotherapy and HT, the patient's condition improved, and he experienced no major side effects within four months. Computerized tomography (CT) revealed no signs of cholangiocarcinoma progression. By raising the tumor's core temperature above 40 °C, ion beam-mediated MHT can stop tumor growth. This suggests that the combination of HT and chemotherapy is a promising pathway for cancer treatment [119].

2.4.1.2 Applications of MNPs in cancer immunotherapeutics

Numerous treatments, known as cancer immunotherapies, use the body's immune system to identify, inhibit, and even target cancer cells easily. Many approaches have been considered to elicit therapeutic immune responses, such as introducing checkpoint drugs based on anti-CTLA-4, anti-PD1/anti-PD-L1 [121], dendritic cell-based vaccines [122], cell transfer methods [123], and combinations [124, 125]. Combining MNPs with cancer immunotherapy techniques yields several advantages and enhances the treatment effect in a specific target area. This combination creates a precisely calibrated delivery vehicle with the necessary surface properties and size to optimize delivery efficiency, which can be guided by a magnetic field. Certain MNP formulations for immunotherapy have been used as *in vivo* MRI contrast agents and fluorescence probes [126]. Gondan *et al* checked the anticancer effect of the polyIC-imiquimod complexes and engineered MNPs in a mouse model for cancer treatment. They demonstrated the potential for clinical trials of vaccines for cancer immunotherapy with these synergistic TLR agonists, MNPs, and immune checkpoint inhibition [124]. Jiang *et al* used MNPs that caused mitochondria-targeted magnetothermal immunogenic cell death to activate tumor-associated macrophages for cancer immunotherapy [127].

2.4.1.3 Use of MNPs for drug delivery in cancer treatment

The primary drawback of the chemotherapy approach is its non-specificity, which damages both healthy and diseased cells. When combined with an external magnetic field, MNPs can overcome this problem by delivering the therapeutic agents to the specified target region and retaining the particles during drug release. Iron oxide MNPs have shown potential for use in drug delivery [128]. The use of MNPs enables particles to be carried to the intended target location, keeps them at that location while the medication is administered, and functions locally (magnetic drug targeting) when combined with an external magnetic field [129]. Medicines might be delivered to a designated area to lessen adverse reactions and the required dosage. To render the particles safe and appropriate for additional functionalization by connecting other bioactive molecules, their surfaces are typically altered using organic polymers and inorganic metals or oxides [130].

2.4.2 Use of MNPs in cancer diagnostics

2.4.2.1 Imaging

State-of-the-art imaging techniques are always used to design imaging systems and increase the efficacy of image capture. These methods include optical fluorescence imaging, ultrasonic imaging, photoacoustic (PA) imaging, CT, MRI, and various others, as shown in figure 2.8 [131, 132]. MRI employs radio waves and strong magnetic fields to produce images of specific organs and tissues [133]. Various types of maps are used in MRI. CT is a method that uses x-rays to produce fine-grained images of blood vessels, soft tissues, bones, and internal organs. The use of ionizing radiation, namely x-rays, is a significant drawback of the CT technique [134].

2.4.2.2 MRI contrast agents

MRI is a visually appealing imaging method and a potent cancer diagnostic tool with outstanding capabilities such as high contrast in soft tissue imaging and great spatial resolution. Nuclear magnetic resonance (NMR) and MRI operate on the same principles. These methods use a strong magnetic field to align the nuclear spins in the patient's body with the direction of the applied magnetic field. A nonequilibrium state is produced when resonant radio-frequency radiation causes the nucleus to absorb energy and raises the spin number to a higher-energy state (in the opposite direction to that of the applied magnetic field). SPIONs have recently been investigated as novel negative contrast agents for MRI image enhancement in T2-weighted images. When exposed to an external magnetic field, MNPs create large gradients in small areas. Because of the susceptibility effects of the iron core, these tiny field gradients provide dark or negative contrast in T2-weighted images and shorten the relaxation times of nuclear spins (T1, T2, and T2*). MNPs should have colloidal stability and low toxicity when used in biological settings for MRI

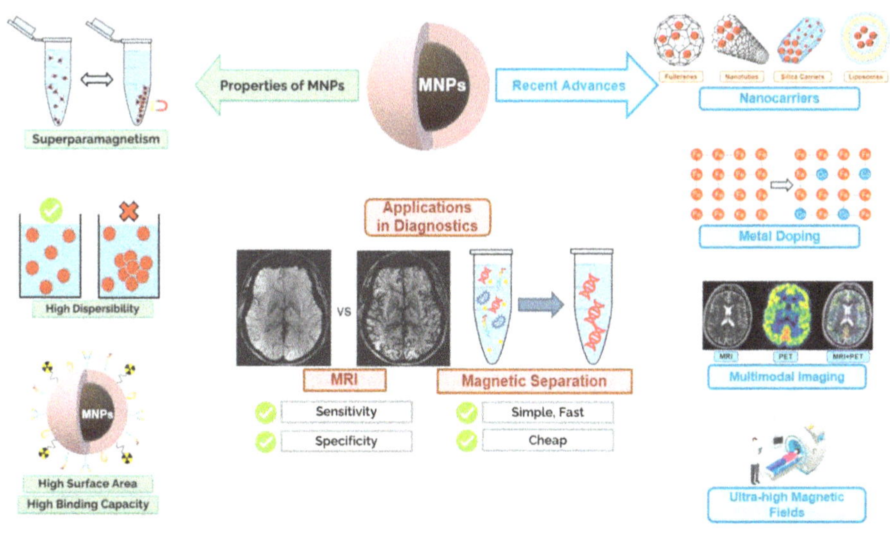

Figure 2.8. Application of MNPs in diagnostics, such as MRI, PET, and MRI–PET. Adapted with permission from [132]. CC BY 4.0.

imaging. When used as contrast agents in MRI, NPs are coated with dextran, dextrin, or protein to accomplish this [133, 135].

Small-sized iron oxide nanoparticles (IONPs) are efficient T1 contrast agents for obtaining good-resolution magnetic resonance angiography in beagle dogs, as shown by Lu *et al.* Kim *et al* showed that the magnetic characteristics of MNPs are strongly affected by particle size. Homogeneous extremely small iron oxide NPs (ESIONs) of varying diameters (1.5, 2.2, 3, and 12 nm) were produced. As the particle size was reduced, the magnetic properties of the synthesized ESIONs generally decreased. In the various forms of the canted precession effect, the spins on the surface molecules are never perfectly aligned. In IONPs 3 nm in size, 93.6% of the particle volume consists of a surface layer 0.8 nm thick where the magnetic spins are canted. In IONPs with diameters of 12 and 2.2 nm, 38.6% and 99.4% of the spins, respectively, are canted. Vessels were clearly evident in T1 MRI after 12 nm ESIONs were inserted into a rat model through its vein, demonstrating that ESIONs can enhance T1 relaxation in the circulatory system [136]. Zho *et al* demonstrated that T1 contrast effects are enhanced when iron NPs are doped with a rare-earth element. They produced iron oxide (GdIO) NPs embedded with gadolinium and evaluated the impact of doping on T1 magnetic resonance contrast [137].

2.4.2.3 Biosensors

Because of their potential to be tuned, MNPs are a viable choice for diagnostic instruments, offering increased sensitivity, comprehensive sampling, and ease of use. MNPs, for instance, can interact with and gather protein samples from various tissues while remaining in the circulatory system. The MNPs can be targeted and even extracted for further examination using magnetic fields. Furthermore, without a proper flow system, MNPs can be used *in vitro* to monitor cell cultures continuously [138, 139]. MNPs employed in biosensors benefit from high magnetism and transverse relaxivity, good surface chemistry that allows for easy modification with binding affinity molecules like peptides, high stability in water solutions to prevent increased aggregation, and superparamagnetic characteristics. Iron core MNPs and ferrite NPs doped with Mn, Co, or Ni have been found to exhibit appropriate characteristics for use in biosensor applications [140, 141].

Manganese-doped ferrite NPs (Mn–MNPs) with a suitable diameter (less than 16 nm), good transverse relaxivity, and high magnetization strength were employed by Lee *et al* for the magnetic particle core. To increase the signal-to-noise ratio (SNR), they coated the NMR probe with tiny molecules of 2,3-dimercaptosuccinic acid. Attaching monoclonal antibodies (against EGFR, EpCAM, or HER2/neu) to the particles' surface allowed Mn–MNP to target cancer cells. Ten antibody molecules were attached to each manufactured particle to improve its hydrodynamic diameter. Under *in vivo* conditions, these compound NPs exhibited sustained stability. Lee *et al* demonstrated that enhanced detection sensitivity was achieved by their designed NMR system and high-strength magnetic Mn-doped ferrite NPs. Single-cell levels ($\approx$2 cells in a 1 μL detection volume) could be detected using the developed NMR system with $MnFe_2O_4$ NPs. These findings attest to this detection technology's great sensitivity and suitability for use in precise biological diagnosis systems [142]. In this study, Proença *et al* [143] used $Co_{0.25}Zn_{0.75}Fe_2O_4$ modified with antibodies to immunocapture CYFRA 21-1 and simulate a peroxidase-like enzyme for amperometric detection. Based on this, a microfluidic system was created to identify CYFRA 21-1, a protein biomarker for prostate cancer. For the first time, $Co_{0.25}Zn_{0.75}Fe_2O_4$ NPs, which have a high magnetic capacity and good biocompatibility when compared to conventional ferrites, were used for biomarker detection [144]. CdSe/CdS/ZnS nanocrystals embellished with Fe_3O_4 NPs were synthesized by Qureshi *et al* for point-of-care optomagnetic detection of cancer biomarkers in serum [145].

2.4.3 Applications of MNPs in biomedical assays

MNP-based methods, such as magnetic separation and magnetic solid-phase extraction, can be used to purify a variety of biomolecules. These methods make separating and purifying target compounds easier without requiring complex chromatographic equipment. Thus, MNPs are frequently employed in biomedical application domains such as protein purification, cell sorting, immunoassay, nucleic acid production, early tumor cell and biomarker identification, and cell, virus, and exosome isolation [146].

The surfaces of MNPs have been altered using a number of functional groups that have the ability to immobilize various biological ligands in an analyte [147]. A primary purpose of commonly used MNPs is to separate and purify analytes. These include histidine-tagged MNPs [148], heparin-tagged MNPs [149], flag-tagged MNPs, and antibody-containing MNPs (protein A/protein G/protein L) [150, 151].

2.4.3.1 Use of MNPs in cell separation

Magnetic-activated cell sorting (MACS) binds MNPs to particular biorecognition molecules during cell separation, including antigens, glycoproteins, and particular structural elements on the cell surface [152, 153], as well as nucleic acid probes, antibiotics, and phages [154]. The target cells are enriched and purified by applying a magnetic field to separate the MNP-tagged cells from the mixtures. Positive and negative sorting approaches comprise most current MNP cell-sorting procedures. Direct and indirect positive sorting are two subcategories of positive sorting. Marking target cells with an initial antibody that is either non-coupled, biotinylated, or fluorescein-coupled is known as indirect positive sorting, which binds to cells using their unique binding properties, affinity, and adsorption properties. These labeled cells are then attached to MNPs through secondary antibodies, such as IgG, anti-biotin–streptavidin, or anti-fluorescein, to facilitate cell separation. On the other hand, during negative sorting, MNPs bind to undesirable cells, leaving the target cells alone. Applications for nanoscale MNPs in cell sorting include cancer research, immunotherapy, and single-cell analysis. MNPs with sizes of less than 250 nm are robust and biocompatible and do not affect a cell's ability to operate physiologically [155]. The US Food and Drug Administration and the EU have approved two systems based on immunomagnetic separation technology for cell separation [156].

2.4.3.2 Use of the MNPs in gene delivery

MNPs employed in the delivery of genes have been coupled to the delivery mechanism and facilitated cellular uptake through their ability to encapsulate genes [157]. Nonviral transfection agents showed a noteworthy advancement in gene transport using novel chemistry and physics-based techniques that are beneficial for energetic processes and charge interactions. This approach works better for gene transfection using biocompatible MNPs *in vivo* and *in vitro*. In the future, MNPs may be attached to the reporter gene utilizing high-field magnets for rapid and excellent transfection of the targeted spot's cells or tissues [158]. NP technology is the most effective technique for directing DNA gene distribution into cells and tissues with regulated assembly behavior. For gene delivery, NPs coated with polyethylenimine have been shown to bind to DNA [159]. The surface modification of iron-oxide-based MNPs improved transfection effectiveness and reduced cytotoxicity during magnetofection. Gene therapy, using a magnetic field to enhance the delivery of therapeutic genes across the blood–brain barrier with minimal toxicity, represents a highly effective method to treat brain tumors. This approach utilizes polyamidoamine dendrimers and magnetosomes conjugated with Tat peptides, which, when exposed to an external magnetic field, facilitate the transport of these gene-carrying nanoparticles into brain tissues. Notably, the incorporation of Tat peptides has shown to improved transfection efficiency. Moreover, gene transfection combined with NP technologies (MNPs) improves the treatment of cancer cells [108, 160].

2.4.3.3 Additional uses of MNPs in disease treatment

MNPs are widely used in deep brain stimulation (DBS), cell treatment, magnetic transfection technology, and the regeneration and repair of injured tissues and organs, in addition to the previously listed biological uses. Only magnetic fields have the ability to physically alter neuronal activity without the need for hardware implants, as they can enter the brain without being absorbed or dispersed [199]. Therefore, a variety of neural modulation techniques using MNPs have been quickly developed to enhance current therapy approaches and offer fresh therapeutic concepts [200]. Magnetothermal and magnetomechanical stimulation are the two most frequently used magnetic DBS techniques. Through the mechanical stimulation that MNSs cause, magnetic nanostructures (MNSs), which are employed in tissue engineering and regenerative medicine, can target stem cells magnetically, promoting cell differentiation. Additionally, the frameworks produced by MNSs improve cell adhesion and proliferation, which raises the frameworks' efficacy *in vivo* and aids in tissue healing [201]. Furthermore, the advantage of a magnetic field may cause mechanical stimulation that activates certain cell surface receptors, upregulating genes linked to growth [202]. According to the discussion above, the various uses of synthesized MNP products include both *in vitro* and *in vivo* applications, including targeted drug delivery, cellular therapy, MHT, medical imaging, cell separation, magnetic transfection, DBS, nucleic acid detection, and magnetic solid-phase extraction technologies, as shown in table 2.2. Because of their unique benefits and widespread use, *in vitro* MNP products have gradually replaced earlier technologies as the preferred option among these applications. Although the

Table 2.2. Examples of selected MNPs, their characteristics, and applications.

S. No.	MNPs	Synthesis method	Characteristics (shape, size, and morphology)	Applications	References
1.	Iron oxide NPs	Alkaline for coprecipitation	10.6 nm, nanospheres	For theranostic applications	[161]
2.	Fe_3O_4@Au nanoroses	Coprecipitation	70 nm flower-like clusters	In combination with MRI, for tumor chemotherapy	[162]
3.	Fe_3O_4–CMCH	Coprecipitation	10 nm, spherical	Drug release and HT treatment for cancer	[163]
4.	Protein-modified Fe_3O_4	Coprecipitation	10 nm, crystalline	Drug delivery in cancer treatment	[164]
5.	PEG–Fe_3O_4	Coprecipitation	25 nm, spherical	Catalytic activity in BPA degradation	[165]
6.	PSS–Fe_3O_4	Coprecipitation	50–200 nm, spherical	Biomedical applications	[166]
7.	IONPs	Alkaline for coprecipitation in a microreactor with hydrodynamic flow focus	24.6 ± 7.1 nm, nanospheres	NMR-based biosensors and MRI	[167]
8.	Ag–MNPs@PCL	Coprecipitation	14–22 nm, spherical	Wound healing application	[168]
9.	Na–citrate/CTAB/TMAH tagged	Coprecipitation method	17–21 nm, spherical	DNA tracer	[169]
10.	PEG–Fe_3O_4	Coprecipitation	25 nm, spherical	Catalysis	[165]
11.	Fe_3O_4 NPs	Hydrothermal	40.16 nm, (pores)	Removal of heavy metal toxicity	[170]
12.	CPPs–CTS@MNPs	Hydrothermal followed by coprecipitation	2–10 nm	Gene delivery	[171]
13.	Pa–M/Ti–NCs	One-pot hydrothermal	80 nm, spherical	Ferroptosis immunomodulation	[172]
14.	MNPs	Hydrothermal synthesis on carbon nanotubes	Solid, hollow, and porous nanospheres	Anode materials in lithium-ion batteries	[3]
15.	Fe_3O_4@TiO_2@Lys MIPs	Sonication	380 nm, spherical	Phosphoprotein biomarker separation	[173]
16.	Strontium oxide NPs	Sonication	43 nm, crystalline	Electrochemical sensors	[174]

(Continued)

Table 2.2. (*Continued*)

S. No.	MNPs	Synthesis method	Characteristics (shape, size, and morphology)	Applications	References
17.	Magnetic oxide NPs	Sonication	N/a	Photothermal therapy, catalysis, direct drug delivery, dual-modality imaging (CT/MRI), and immunoassays	[175]
18.	Fe_3O_4@C/Ag Nps	Solvothermal	360–733 nm, spherical	Dye degradation	[176]
19.	Fe_3O_4	Solvothermal and heat treatment	Thickness: 50 nm, inner diameter: 800 nm, outer diameter: 5 μm.	Electromagnetic applications	[177]
20.	Fe_3O_4	Solvothermal	10–150 nm, anti-spinel.	Water treatment	[178]
21.	Ferrite (Mn, Co, and Zn) NPs	Thermal decomposition	Diameter: 3–5 nm, crystalline	N/a	[45]
22.	Magnetite NPs	Thermal decomposition	10–29 nm, spherical	Biomedical applications	[179]
23.	$CoFe_2O_4$	Thermal decomposition	Na	Catalysis	[180]
24.	(MFe_2O_4, M = Fe^{2+}, Ni^{2+}, Mn^{2+}, Co^{2+}, Zn^{2+})	Spray pyrolysis	Diameters:121.13, 43.19, 33.21, 33.28, and 33.63 nm.	Cancer treatment	[181]
25.	Cu-based MNPs.	Pyrolysis	Diameter: 2.8 nm	Cancer treatment, contrast agent	[182]
26.	$Mn_{0.25}Mg_{0.25}Co_{0.5}Fe_2O_4$	Sol–gel	32 nm, cubic	Antibacterial applications and cancer treatment	[183]
27.	$La_{0.6}Sr_{0.4}MnO_3$	Sol–gel	N/a	HT application	[184]
28.	SiO_2–CaO–Na_2O–P_2O_5	Sol–gel	Particle sizes: 2, 15, 18, and 43 nm, spherical.	Magnetic fluid CT, employed in HT treatment	[185]
29.	Palladium NPs	Microwave-assisted synthesis	5–30 nm, brown, spherical morphology.	Photocatalytic and biomedical applications	[186]
30.	Usnic acid-loaded magnetite NPs	Microwave-assisted hydrothermal method	N/a	Anticancer treatments	[187]

31.	IONPs.	Microwave-assisted synthesis	Crystallite size of 9 nm	MRI contrast agent, thermal mediator in HT, and integrated into drug delivery systems	[188]
32.	Silver NPs	Microwave-assisted green synthesis	171.81 nm, crystalline structure	Biologically active agent, carrier for drug delivery	[189]
33.	MNPs	Microwave treatment	N/a	Liver cancer treatment	[190]
34.	Superparamagnetic NPs	Microemulsion	Diameters between 5.4 and 7.2 nm	Analytical applications	[191]
35.	Silica-coated Fe_3O_4.	Microemulsion	16 ± 0.14 nm, cubic	Antimicrobial activity	[192]
36.	Au NPs	Microemulsion	19–40 nm, spherical	Biomedical applications	[193]
37.	Bacteria-based MNPs	Biological	40.6 ± 7.2 nm	MHT therapy	[194]
38.	IONPs	Biological	10–40 nm, spherical	Cancer treatments	[195]
39.	$Mn_{0.5}Zn_{0.5}Er_xY_xFe_{2-2x}O_4$	Ultrasonic	N/a	Biomedical applications	[196]
40.	MNPs	Ultrasonic	Diameter: 50 nm	MHT therapy	[197]
41.	$Mn_{0.5}Zn_{0.5}Fe_2O_4$ nanoflowers	Hydrothermal	N/a	Magnetic fluid HT	[198]

PSS (polystyrene sulfonic acid), CTAB (hyexadecyltrimethylammonium bromide), TMAH (tetra methyl ammonium hydroxide), BPA (bisphenyol A), CPP-CTS@ MNPs(cell penetrating peptide conjugated chitosan modified iron oxide magnetic nanoparticles).

results are clear for *in vivo* applications, MNP products can still only be used for a small number of applications because of lengthy clinical trial periods.

2.5 Hybrid MNPs and overall industrial manufacture

To overcome the drawbacks of single-component NPs, enhance their properties, introduce new capabilities unattainable by individual components, and enable multifunctionality within a single nanoframework, research has shifted toward the development of hybrid nanostructures. These structures are composed of at least two different materials. Various hybrid nanostructures have been designed and fabricated, such as core–shell and yolk–shell configurations, heterodimers, Janus particles, dot-in-nanotubes, dot-on-nanorods, and nanobranches. These structures exhibit controlled magnetic properties by incorporating iron, cobalt, zinc, manganese–ferrite, or mixed ferrites [203–207] Numerous material pairings, including plasmonic/catalytic, magnetic/luminescent, and catalytic, have been tried successfully, greatly increasing the collection of useful materials and possibly spawning new study fields such as plasmon-enhanced photovoltaics [208, 209] and plasmon-enhanced photocatalysis.

These MNPs have diverse biomedical applications. Hybrid NPs (HNPs) need to be surface functionalized in most biomedical applications and to benefit from the advantages of functionalization. HNPs are typically coated with an inorganic or organic coating to produce water-soluble colloids because the synthesis techniques typically used to create HNPs result in hydrophobic particles. For instance, a carbon coating can be applied to Fe and Co particles with unusually high magnetization to make them chemically stable and biocompatible [210], or a reverse microemulsion technique can be used to coat iron oxides with a thin SiO_2 shell [211]. As an alternative, organic molecules can coat HNPs to provide stability in water, and single-phase MNPs can also be surface functionalized [212]. The most widely used tactics swap out oleate molecules for hydrophilic ones such as methoxy poly (ethylene glycol), citrate [213], various hydroxides [203], dopamine-containing polymers, or others [214]. An alternative is to cover the oleate-coated HNPs with polymers containing hydrophilic and hydrophobic groups, preserving the original ligands while offering more functionalization choices. On previously created Au NPs, $Fe(CO)_5$ was broken down in 1-octadecene and oleic acid to create hybrid iron-oxide–metal nanostructures [215]. By creating Au/Fe MNP oxide interfaces, this process produced NPs with a Janus (two-faced) structure, minimal polydispersity, and a comparatively low lattice mismatch. Alternatively, Ag/Fe_3O_4 nanoflowers, which were created using a single-step solvothermal technique and comprised Ag domains encased in aggregated Fe_3O_4 nanocrystals [216], exhibited improved optical and magnetic absorption. Research by Guardia *et al* examined the properties of Au/Fe NP oxide dimers in cancer treatment by performing HT experiments; they found that chloride ions could help the assembly of the Fe on the surface of the gold NPs [216]. Recently, Curcio *et al* [217] showed that CuS shells may be applied to iron oxide HNP nanoflowers made using the polyol method [218], allowing for a significant photothermal conversion application of infrared light. This method of production relies on cupric nitrate reacting with polyvinylpyrrolidone and hydrazine to generate a Cu_2O shell on the NPs. In a second step, the NPs are treated with ammonium sulfide. The oxide is then sulfated, and a spiky CuS shell is formed.

2.5.1 Application of hybrid MNPs in cancer theranostics

HNPs offer an additional degree of flexibility that can be used to customize their overall characteristics and achieve some of the highest values ever recorded [203, 219]. The inherent drawbacks of traditional single-phase nanomaterials can be addressed using HNPs. For instance, the HNP architecture can encourage incoherent reversal modes and regulate the effective operation of HNPs without altering the total particle size [203, 220]. Bi-magnetic core/shell $CoFe_2O_4/MnFe_2O_4$ has been reported to be more effective than Feridex and doxorubicin at killing U87MG cancer cell lines in a nude mouse model when used as a HT treatment. The cubic shape of $MnFe_2O_4/CoFe_2O_4$ core/shell NPs allows for more effective HT treatment of drug-resistant cancer cells [221, 222]. $Zn_{0.4}Co_{0.6}$–Fe_2O_4 MNPs coupled with Zn (II)-bis(dipicolylamine) (bis-ZnDPA) and a chemotherapeutic medication (b-Lap) demonstrated a superior MHT function that suppressed tumor development and self-amplified apoptosis targeting [223]. HNPs that mix optical and magnetic components have drawn much interest from theranostics researchers because of their unique multifunctional qualities, ranging from imaging and diagnosis to treatment [224]. Numerous investigations, particularly using Fe_3O_4/Au nanostructures, have demonstrated improved dual heating efficiency using simultaneous alternating magnetic fields and laser irradiation [225, 226]. In contrast, magnetic-field-guided photothermal treatment has been employed with Au/Fe_3O_4 NPs [227, 228]. Besides being a regulated anticancer drug vehicle, Au-tagged or coated Fe_3O_4 NPs demonstrated an improved photothermal response [229]. Fan *et al* used aptamer-coupled Fe_3O_4/Au NPs to demonstrate targeted diagnosis, separation, and irreversible cancer cell destruction after 10 min of exposure to 670 nm light at 2.5 W cm^2 [230]. It has recently been demonstrated that magnetic–plasmonic Fe_3O_4/Au significantly improved glioma cell treatment [231]. The photothermal efficiency of PEGylated Fe/Fe_3O_4 HNPs was similar to that of Au nanorods. Dual-mode magnetic resonance and computed tomography imaging has also been carried out using magneto-plasmonic Fe_3O_4/Au NPs [232, 233].

References

[1] Zhou K, Zhou X, Liu J and Huang Z 2020 Application of magnetic nanoparticles in petroleum industry: a review *J. Petrol. Sci. Eng.* **188** 106943

[2] Nkurikiyimfura I, Wang Y, Safari B and Nshingabigwi E 2020 Temperature-dependent magnetic properties of magnetite nanoparticles synthesized via coprecipitation method *J. Alloys Compd.* **846** 156344

[3] Niculescu A-G, Chircov C and Grumezescu A M 2022 Magnetite nanoparticles: synthesis methods–a comparative review *Methods* **199** 16–27

[4] Samrot A V, Sahithya C S, Selvarani J, Purayil S K and Ponnaiah P 2021 A review on synthesis, characterization and potential biological applications of superparamagnetic iron oxide nanoparticles *Curr. Res. Green Sustain. Chem.* **4** 100042

[5] Setia A, Mehata A K, Malik A K, Viswanadh M K and Muthu M S 2023 Theranostic magnetic nanoparticles: synthesis, properties, toxicity, and emerging trends for biomedical applications *J. Drug Deliv. Sci. Technol.* **81** 104295

[6] Shen B and Sun S 2020 Chemical synthesis of magnetic nanoparticles for permanent magnet applications *Chem.–A Eur. J.* **26** 6757–66

[7] Dave S, Dave S, Mathur A and Das J 2021 Biological synthesis of magnetic nanoparticles *Nanobiotechnology* (Amsterdam: Elsevier) pp 225–34

[8] Majidi S, Zeinali Sehrig F, Farkhani S M, Soleymani Goloujeh M and Akbarzadeh A 2016 Current methods for synthesis of magnetic nanoparticles *Artif. Cells, Nanomed. Biotechnol.* **44** 722–34

[9] Ziarani G M, Malmir M, Lashgari N and Badiei A 2019 The role of hollow magnetic nanoparticles in drug delivery *RSC Adv.* **9** 25094–106

[10] Sun Y, Li H, Cui G, Wu X, Yang M, Piao Y, Bai Z, Wang L, Kraft M and Zhao W 2022 A magnetic nanoparticle assisted microfluidic system for low abundance cell sorting with high recovery *Micro Nano Eng.* **15** 100136

[11] Zhang X, Wang Z, Xie H, Sun R, Cao T, Paudyal N, Fang W and Song H 2018 Development of a magnetic nanoparticles-based screen-printed electrodes (MNPs-SPEs) biosensor for the quantification of ochratoxin A in cereal and feed samples *Toxins* **10** 317

[12] Felton C, Karmakar A, Gartia Y, Ramidi P, Biris A S and Ghosh A 2014 Magnetic nanoparticles as contrast agents in biomedical imaging: recent advances in iron-and manganese-based magnetic nanoparticles *Drug Metab. Rev.* **46** 142–54

[13] Makridis A, Topouridou K, Tziomaki M, Sakellari D, Simeonidis K, Angelakeris M, Yavropoulou M P, Yovos J G and Kalogirou O 2014 *In vitro* application of Mn-ferrite nanoparticles as novel magnetic hyperthermia agents *J. Mater. Chem.* B **2** 8390–8

[14] Farzin A, Etesami S A, Quint J, Memic A and Tamayol A 2020 Magnetic nanoparticles in cancer therapy and diagnosis *Adv. Healthc. Mater.* **9** 1901058

[15] Rezaei B, Yari P, Sanders S M, Wang H, Chugh V K, Liang S, Mostufa S, Xu K, Wang J P and Gómez-Pastora J 2024 Magnetic nanoparticles: a review on synthesis, characterization, functionalization, and biomedical applications *Small* **20** 2304848

[16] Kruis F E, Fissan H and Peled A 1998 Synthesis of nanoparticles in the gas phase for electronic, optical and magnetic applications—a review *J. Aerosol Sci.* **29** 511–35

[17] Stiufiuc G F and Stiufiuc R I 2024 Magnetic nanoparticles: synthesis, characterization, and their use in biomedical field *Appl. Sci.* **14** 1623

[18] Mattox D M 2000 Ion plating—past, present and future *Surf. Coat. Technol.* **133** 517–21

[19] Sun S-N, Wei C, Zhu Z-Z, Hou Y-L, Venkatraman S S and Xu Z-C 2014 Magnetic iron oxide nanoparticles: synthesis and surface coating techniques for biomedical applications *Chin. Phys.* B **23** 037503

[20] Mosayebi J, Kiyasatfar M and Laurent S 2017 Synthesis, functionalization, and design of magnetic nanoparticles for theranostic applications *Adv. Healthc. Mater.* **6** 1700306

[21] Rane A V, Kanny K, Abitha V and Thomas S 2018 Methods for synthesis of nanoparticles and fabrication of nanocomposites *Synthesis of Inorganic Nanomaterials* (Amsterdam: Elsevier) pp 121–39

[22] Hammad M, Hardt S, Mues B, Salamon S, Landers J, Slabu I, Wende H, Schulz C and Wiggers H 2020 Gas-phase synthesis of iron oxide nanoparticles for improved magnetic hyperthermia performance *J. Alloys Compd.* **824** 153814
[23] Corbierre M K, Beerens J and Lennox R B 2005 Gold nanoparticles generated by electron beam lithography of gold (I)-thiolate thin films *Chem. Mater.* **17** 5774–9
[24] Tseng A A, Chen K, Chen C D and Ma K J 2003 Electron beam lithography in nanoscale fabrication: recent development *IEEE Trans. Electron. Packag. Manuf.* **26** 141–9
[25] Jia C-J, Sun L-D, Luo F, Han X-D, Heyderman L J, Yan Z-G, Yan C-H, Zheng K, Zhang Z and Takano M 2008 Large-scale synthesis of single-crystalline iron oxide magnetic nanorings *JACS* **130** 16968–77
[26] Lv B, Liu Z, Tian H, Xu Y, Wu D and Sun Y 2010 Single-crystalline dodecahedral and octodecahedralα-Fe_2O_3 particles synthesized by a fluoride anion–assisted hydrothermal method *Adv. Funct. Mater.* **20** 3987–96
[27] Willmott P and Huber J 2000 Pulsed laser vaporization and deposition *Rev. Mod. Phys.* **72** 315
[28] Gavrila-Florescu L, Dumitrache F, Balas M, Fleaca C T, Scarisoreanu M, Morjan I P, Dutu E, Ilie A, Banici A-M and Locovei C 2017 Synthesis of Fe-based core@ ZnO shell nanopowders by laser pyrolysis for biomedical applications *Appl. Phys.* A **123** 1–13
[29] Kongkaew S, Srilikhit A, Janduang S, Thipwimonmas Y, Kanatharana P, Thavarungkul P and Limbut W 2024 Single laser synthesis of gold nanoparticles-polypyrrole-chitosan on laser-induced graphene for ascorbic acid detection *Talanta* **278** 126446
[30] Alonso J, Barandiarán J M, Barquín L F and García-Arribas A 2018 Magnetic nanoparticles, synthesis, properties, and applications *Magnetic Nanostructured Materials* (Amsterdam: Elsevier) pp 1–40
[31] Arbain R, Othman M and Palaniandy S 2011 Preparation of iron oxide nanoparticles by mechanical milling *Miner. Eng.* **24** 1–9
[32] Chen B W, Hatamie S, Garu P, Heravi P, Chen J Y, Liu B T, Wei Z H and Yao D J 2020 Synthesis of iron-oxide magnetic nanoparticles coated with dextran of varied molecular mass using a facile ball-milling method *Micro Nano Lett.* **15** 645–50
[33] Velásquez A and Urquijo J 2021 Synthesis and characterization of magnetite–maghemite nanoparticles in presence of polyethylene glycol obtained by mechanical milling *Mater. Sci. Eng.:* B **263** 114873
[34] Wirunchit S, Gansa P and Koetniyom W 2021 Synthesis of ZnO nanoparticles by Ball-milling process for biological applications *Mater. Today Proc.* **47** 3554–9
[35] Darr J A, Zhang J, Makwana N M and Weng X 2017 Continuous hydrothermal synthesis of inorganic nanoparticles: applications and future directions *Chem. Rev.* **117** 11125–238
[36] Das B and Mohanty S 2024 A comprehensive review on piezoelectric inks: from concept to application *Sens. Actuators,* A **366** 114939
[37] Kurian J, Lahiri B, Mathew M J and Philip J 2021 High magnetic fluid hyperthermia efficiency in copper ferrite nanoparticles prepared by solvothermal and hydrothermal methods *J. Magn. Magn. Mater.* **538** 168233
[38] Fotukian S M, Barati A, Soleymani M and Alizadeh A M 2020 Solvothermal synthesis of $CuFe_2O_4$ and Fe_3O_4 nanoparticles with high heating efficiency for magnetic hyperthermia application *J. Alloys Compd.* **816** 152548
[39] Pathak S, Verma R, Singhal S, Chaturvedi R, Kumar P, Sharma P, Pant R P and Wang X 2021 Spin dynamics investigations of multifunctional ambient scalable Fe_3O_4 surface decorated ZnO magnetic nanocomposite using FMR *Sci. Rep.* **11** 3799

[40] Faraji M, Yamini Y and Rezaee M 2010 Magnetic nanoparticles: synthesis, stabilization, functionalization, characterization, and applications *J. Iran. Chem. Soc.* **7** 1–37
[41] Kim D, Zhang Y, Voit W, Rao K and Muhammed M 2001 Synthesis and characterization of surfactant-coated superparamagnetic monodispersed iron oxide nanoparticles *J. Magn. Magn. Mater.* **225** 30–6
[42] Houshiar M, Zebhi F, Razi Z J, Alidoust A and Askari Z 2014 Synthesis of cobalt ferrite ($CoFe_2O_4$) nanoparticles using combustion, coprecipitation, and precipitation methods: a comparison study of size, structural, and magnetic properties *J. Magn. Magn. Mater.* **371** 43–8
[43] Saremi A, Mirkazemi S M, Sazvar A and Rezaie H 2024 Controlling magnetic and surface properties of cobalt ferrite nanoparticles: a comparison of co-precipitation and solvothermal synthesis methods *Solid State Sci.* **148** 107432
[44] Muni Babu B, Sivakumar R and Sanjeeviraja C 2022 Studies on the properties of copper tin hydroxide-based catalysts prepared by co-precipitation method for photocatalytic degradation of methylene blue dye *J. Mater. Sci., Mater. Electron.* **33** 11687–700
[45] Ivanova A, Ivanova E, Nikitin A, Cherepanov V and Abakumov M 2024 Thermal decomposition of acetylacetonates for highly reproducible synthesis of M-ferrite (Mn, Co and Zn) nanoparticles with tunable magnetic properties *J. Alloys Compd.* **976** 172737
[46] Gonzales-Weimuller M, Zeisberger M and Krishnan K M 2009 Size-dependant heating rates of iron oxide nanoparticles for magnetic fluid hyperthermia *J. Magn. Magn. Mater.* **321** 1947–50
[47] Hyeon T, Lee S S, Park J, Chung Y and Na H B 2001 Synthesis of highly crystalline and monodisperse maghemite nanocrystallites without a size-selection process *J. Am. Chem. Soc.* **123** 12798–801
[48] Li X, Wei J, Aifantis K E, Fan Y, Feng Q, Cui F Z and Watari F 2016 Current investigations into magnetic nanoparticles for biomedical applications *J. Biomed. Mater. Res.* A **104** 1285–96
[49] Kim D, Shin K, Kwon S G and Hyeon T 2018 Synthesis and biomedical applications of multifunctional nanoparticles *Adv. Mater.* **30** 1802309
[50] Liu S, Yu B, Wang S, Shen Y and Cong H 2020 Preparation, surface functionalization and application of Fe_3O_4 magnetic nanoparticles *Adv. Colloid Interface Sci.* **281** 102165
[51] Endla P 2024 Structure, morphology, and luminescence properties of sol–gel-synthesized pure and cobalt-doped MgO nanoparticles *Ionics* **30** 7653–63
[52] Moradnia F, Fardood S T, Ramazani A, Min B-k, Joo S W and Varma R S 2021 Magnetic $Mg_{0.5}Zn_{0.5}FeMnO_4$ nanoparticles: green sol–gel synthesis, characterization, and photocatalytic applications *J. Clean. Prod.* **288** 125632
[53] Esmaeilkhanian A, Sharifianjazi F, Parvin N and Kooti M A 2021 Cytotoxicity of thermoresponsive core/shell $Ni_xCo_{1-x}Fe_2O_4$/PEG nanoparticles synthesized by the sol–gel method *J. Phys. D: Appl. Phys.* **54** 295002
[54] Onwudiwe D C 2019 Microwave-assisted synthesis of PbS nanostructures *Heliyon* **5** e01413
[55] Brollo M E F, Veintemillas-Verdaguer S, Salván C M and Morales M d P 2017 Key parameters on the microwave assisted synthesis of magnetic nanoparticles for MRI contrast agents *Contrast Media Mol. Imaging* **2017** 8902424
[56] López Y C and Antuch M 2020 Morphology control in the plant-mediated synthesis of magnetite nanoparticles *Curr. Opin. Green Sustain. Chem.* **24** 32–7

[57] Sánchez-López E, Gomes D, Esteruelas G, Bonilla L, Lopez-Machado A L, Galindo R, Cano A, Espina M, Ettcheto M and Camins A 2020 Metal-based nanoparticles as antimicrobial agents: an overview *Nanomaterials* **10** 292
[58] Marcelo G A, Lodeiro C, Capelo J L, Lorenzo J and Oliveira E 2020 Magnetic, fluorescent and hybrid nanoparticles: from synthesis to application in biosystems *Mater. Sci. Eng.* C **106** 110104
[59] Mihai A D, Chircov C, Grumezescu A M and Holban A M 2020 Magnetite nanoparticles and essential oils systems for advanced antibacterial therapies *Int. J. Mol. Sci.* **21** 7355
[60] Jamkhande P G, Ghule N W, Bamer A H and Kalaskar M G 2019 Metal nanoparticles synthesis: an overview on methods of preparation, advantages and disadvantages, and applications *J. Drug Deliv. Sci. Technol.* **53** 101174
[61] Moon J-W, Rawn C J, Rondinone A J, Love L J, Roh Y, Everett S M, Lauf R J and Phelps T J 2010 Large-scale production of magnetic nanoparticles using bacterial fermentation *J. Ind. Microbiol. Biotechnol.* **37** 1023–31
[62] Prabhu N 2018 Green synthesis of iron oxide nanoparticles (IONPs) and their nanotechnological applications *J. Bacteriol. Mycol. Open Access* **6** 260–2
[63] Elblbesy M A-A, Madbouly A K and Hamdan T A-A 2014 Bio-synthesis of magnetite nanoparticles by bacteria *Am. J. Nano Res. Appl.* **2** 98–103
[64] Madubuonu N, Aisida S O, Ali A, Ahmad I, Zhao T-k, Botha S, Maaza M and Ezema F I 2019 Biosynthesis of iron oxide nanoparticles via a composite of *Psidium guavaja-Moringa oleifera* and their antibacterial and photocatalytic study *J. Photochem. Photobiol.*, B **199** 111601
[65] Pierce D E, Wright P J and Popelka-Filcoff R S 2020 Seeing red: an analysis of archeological hematite in east central Missouri *Archaeol. Anthropol. Sci.* **12** 1–20
[66] Samrot A V, Senthilkumar P, Rashmitha S, Veera P and Sahithya C S 2018 Azadirachta indica influenced biosynthesis of super-paramagnetic iron-oxide nanoparticles and their applications in tannery water treatment and X-ray imaging *J. Nanostruct. Chem.* **8** 343–51
[67] Liu J, Wu K and Wang J-P 2024 Physical methods for the synthesis of MNPs *Magnetic Nanoparticles in Nanomedicine* (Amsterdam: Elsevier) pp 83–114
[68] Orellana C, González-Fuentes C, Abellan M, Segura R, Oyarzún S, Acevedo C and Romero C 2024 Spontaneous self-assembly of magnetic nanoparticle chains, at the first stage of a gas aggregation source *Plasma Processes Polym.* **21** e2400002
[69] Taha T, Azab A and Sebak M 2019 Glycerol-assisted sol–gel synthesis, optical, and magnetic properties of $NiFe_2O_4$ nanoparticles *J. Mol. Struct.* **1181** 14–8
[70] Salah N, Habib S S, Khan Z H, Memic A, Azam A, Alarfaj E, Zahed N and Al-Hamedi S 2011 High-energy ball milling technique for ZnO nanoparticles as antibacterial material *Int. J. Nanomed.* **6** 863–9
[71] Klencsár Z, Ábrahám A, Szabó L, Szabó E G, Stichleutner S, Kuzmann E, Homonnay Z and Tolnai G 2019 The effect of preparation conditions on magnetite nanoparticles obtained via chemical co-precipitation *Mater. Chem. Phys.* **223** 122–32
[72] Rodríguez-Rodríguez A A, Moreno-Trejo M B, Meléndez-Zaragoza M J, Collins-Martínez V, López-Ortiz A, Martínez-Guerra E and Sánchez-Domínguez M 2019 Spinel-type ferrite nanoparticles: synthesis by the oil-in-water microemulsion reaction method and photocatalytic water-splitting evaluation *Int. J. Hydrogen Energy* **44** 12421–9
[73] Leonel L V, Barbosa J B, Miquita D R, Oliveira F P, Fernandez-Outon L E, Oliveira E F and Ardisson J D 2018 Facile polyol synthesis of ultrasmall water-soluble cobalt ferrite nanoparticles *Solid State Sci.* **86** 45–52

[74] Andrade R G, Veloso S R and Castanheira E M 2020 Shape anisotropic iron oxide-based magnetic nanoparticles: synthesis and biomedical applications *Int. J. Mol. Sci.* **21** 2455
[75] Zhang H, Lizana A, Iemmi C, Monroy-Ramírez F A, Márquez A, Moreno I and Campos J 2018 LCoS display phase self-calibration method based on diffractive lens schemes *Opt. Lasers Eng.* **106** 147–54
[76] Calderón-Jiménez B, Montoro Bustos A R, Pereira Reyes R, Paniagua S A and Vega-Baudrit J R 2022 Novel pathway for the sonochemical synthesis of silver nanoparticles with near-spherical shape and high stability in aqueous media *Sci. Rep.* **12** 882
[77] Nyabadza A, McCarthy É, Makhesana M, Heidarinassab S, Plouze A, Vazquez M and Brabazon D 2023 A review of physical, chemical and biological synthesis methods of bimetallic nanoparticles and applications in sensing, water treatment, biomedicine, catalysis and hydrogen storage *Adv. Colloid Interface Sci.* **321** 103010
[78] Jawad A S and Al-Alawy A F 2020 Synthesis and characterization of coated magnetic nanoparticles and its application as coagulant for removal of oil droplets from oilfield produced water *AIP Conf. Proc.* **2213** 020174
[79] Mohammadi F, Esrafili A, Sobhi H R, Behbahani M, Kermani M, Asgari E and Fasih Z R 2018 Evaluation of adsorption and removal of methylparaben from aqueous solutions using amino-functionalized magnetic nanoparticles as an efficient adsorbent: optimization and modeling by response surface methodology (RSM) *Desalin. Water Treat.* **103** 248–60
[80] Khan R, Saxena A and Shukla S 2020 Evaluation of heavy metal pollution for River Gomti, in parts of Ganga Alluvial Plain, India *SN Appl. Sci.* **2** 1451
[81] Punia P, Naagar M, Chalia S, Dhar R, Ravelo B, Thakur P and Thakur A 2021 Recent advances in synthesis, characterization, and applications of nanoparticles for contaminated water treatment—a review *Ceram. Int.* **47** 1526–50
[82] Zamani Kouhpanji M R and Stadler B J 2020 A guideline for effectively synthesizing and characterizing magnetic nanoparticles for advancing nanobiotechnology: a review *Sensors* **20** 2554
[83] Galloway J M, Talbot J E, Critchley K, Miles J J and Bramble J P 2015 Developing biotemplated data storage: room temperature biomineralization of L10 CoPt magnetic nanoparticles *Adv. Funct. Mater.* **25** 4590–600
[84] Gabbasov R, Polikarpov M, Cherepanov V, Chuev M, Mischenko I, Lomov A, Wang A and Panchenko V 2015 Mössbauer, magnetization and X-ray diffraction characterization methods for iron oxide nanoparticles *J. Magn. Magn. Mater.* **380** 111–6
[85] Chekli L, Bayatsarmadi B, Sekine R, Sarkar B, Shen A M, Scheckel K, Skinner W, Naidu R, Shon H and Lombi E 2016 Analytical characterisation of nanoscale zero-valent iron: a methodological review *Anal. Chim. Acta* **903** 13–35
[86] Liu Z, Chen G, Xu L, Hu F and Duan X 2019 Removal of Cr (VI) from wastewater by a novel adsorbent of magnetic goethite: adsorption performance and adsorbent characterisation *ChemistrySelect* **4** 13817–27
[87] Reddy L H, Arias J L, Nicolas J and Couvreur P 2012 Magnetic nanoparticles: design and characterization, toxicity and biocompatibility, pharmaceutical and biomedical applications *Chem. Rev.* **112** 5818–78
[88] Yadav V K, Ali D, Khan S H, Gnanamoorthy G, Choudhary N, Yadav K K, Thai V N, Hussain S A and Manhrdas S 2020 Synthesis and characterization of amorphous iron oxide nanoparticles by the sonochemical method and their application for the remediation of heavy metals from wastewater *Nanomaterials* **10** 1551

[89] Ukhurebor K E, Aigbe U O, Onyancha R B, Balogun V A, Anani O A, Adama K K, Pal K, Kusuma H S and Darmokoesoemo H 2023 An overview of magnetic nanomaterials *Magnetic Nanomaterials: Synthesis, Characterization and Applications* (Cham: Springer) pp 1–20

[90] Ida H, Segawa T, Tohyama S and Kawai J 2005 Analysis of painted steel by a hand-held X-ray fluorescence spectrometer *Spectrochim. Acta* B **60** 249–52

[91] Karabelli D, Üzüm C A R, Shahwan T, Eroglu A E, Scott T B, Hallam K R and Lieberwirth I 2008 Batch removal of aqueous Cu^{2+} ions using nanoparticles of zero-valent iron: a study of the capacity and mechanism of uptake *Ind. Eng. Chem. Res.* **47** 4758–64

[92] Löwa N, Fabert J-M, Gutkelch D, Paysen H, Kosch O and Wiekhorst F 2019 3D-printing of novel magnetic composites based on magnetic nanoparticles and photopolymers *J. Magn. Magn. Mater.* **469** 456–60

[93] Zahid M, Nadeem N, Hanif M A, Bhatti I A, Bhatti H N and Mustafa G 2019 Metal ferrites and their graphene-based nanocomposites: synthesis, characterization, and applications in wastewater treatment *Magnetic Nanostructures: Environmental and Agricultural Applications* (Cham: Springer) pp 181–212

[94] Comrie J P 2011 *Molecular Self-assembly: Advances in Chemistry, Biology, and Nanotechnology* (Hauppauge, NY: Nova Science Publishers)

[95] Yi C, Liu H, Zhang S, Yang Y, Zhang Y, Lu Z, Kumacheva E and Nie Z 2020 Self-limiting directional nanoparticle bonding governed by reaction stoichiometry *Science* **369** 1369–74

[96] Nie Z, Petukhova A and Kumacheva E 2010 Properties and emerging applications of self-assembled structures made from inorganic nanoparticles *Nat. Nanotechnol.* **5** 15–25

[97] Ganguly R and Puri I K 2007 Field-assisted self-assembly of superparamagnetic nanoparticles for biomedical, MEMS and BioMEMS applications *Adv. Appl. Mech.* **41** 293–335

[98] Mahmood A U and Yingling Y G 2022 All-atom simulation method for Zeeman alignment and dipolar assembly of magnetic nanoparticles *J. Chem. Theory Comput.* **18** 3122–35

[99] Lalatonne Y, Richardi J and Pileni M 2004 Van der Waals versus dipolar forces controlling mesoscopic organizations of magnetic nanocrystals *Nat. Mater.* **3** 121–5

[100] Neugebauer N, Fabian A, Elm M T, Hofmann D M, Czerner M, Heiliger C and Klar P J 2020 Investigation of the dipole interaction in and between ordered arrangements of magnetic nanoparticles *Phys. Rev.* B **101** 104409

[101] Tian B, Han Y, Fock J, Strömberg M, Leifer K and Hansen M F 2019 Self-assembled magnetic nanoparticle–graphene oxide nanotag for optomagnetic detection of DNA *ACS Appl. Nano Mater.* **2** 1683–90

[102] Konuk E Y 2024 A meta-analysis assessing the cytotoxicity of nanoparticles on MCF7 breast cancer cells *Oncol. Lett.* **28** 551

[103] Vargas R, Lizano-Barrantes C, Romero M, Valencia-Clua K, Narváez-Narváez D A, Suñé-Negre J M, Pérez-Lozano P, García-Montoya E, Martinez-Martinez N and Hernández-Munain C 2024 The piper at the gates of brain: a systematic review of surface modification strategies on lipid nanoparticles to overcome the blood-brain-barrier *Int. J. Pharm.* **665** 124686

[104] Nam J, Son S, Park K S, Zou W, Shea L D and Moon J J 2019 Cancer nanomedicine for combination cancer immunotherapy *Nat. Rev. Mater.* **4** 398–414

[105] Gong F, Yang N, Wang X, Zhao Q, Chen Q, Liu Z and Cheng L 2020 Tumor microenvironment-responsive intelligent nanoplatforms for cancer theranostics *Nano Today* **32** 100851

[106] Chen H, Zhang W, Zhu G, Xie J and Chen X 2017 Rethinking cancer nanotheranostics *Nat. Rev. Mater.* **2** 1–18

[107] Overchuk M and Zheng G 2018 Overcoming obstacles in the tumor microenvironment: recent advancements in nanoparticle delivery for cancer theranostics *Biomaterials* **156** 217–37

[108] Zhao S, Yu X, Qian Y, Chen W and Shen J 2020 Multifunctional magnetic iron oxide nanoparticles: an advanced platform for cancer theranostics *Theranostics* **10** 6278

[109] Liu X, Zhang Y, Wang Y, Zhu W, Li G, Ma X, Zhang Y, Chen S, Tiwari S and Shi K 2020 Comprehensive understanding of magnetic hyperthermia for improving antitumor therapeutic efficacy *Theranostics* **10** 3793

[110] Roy I 2022 Therapeutic applications of magnetic nanoparticles: recent advances *Mater. Adv.* **3** 7425–44

[111] Pathak S, Jain K, Kumar P, Wang X and Pant R P 2019 Improved thermal performance of annular fin-shell tube storage system using magnetic fluid *Appl. Energy* **239** 1524–35

[112] Beik J, Abed Z, Ghoreishi F S, Hosseini-Nami S, Mehrzadi S, Shakeri-Zadeh A and Kamrava S K 2016 Nanotechnology in hyperthermia cancer therapy: from fundamental principles to advanced applications *J. Control. Release* **235** 205–21

[113] Szwed M and Marczak A 2024 Application of nanoparticles for magnetic hyperthermia for cancer treatment—the current state of knowledge *Cancers* **16** 1156

[114] Rahban D, Doostan M and Salimi A 2020 Cancer therapy; prospects for application of nanoparticles for magnetic-based hyperthermia *Cancer Invest.* **38** 507–21

[115] Lanier O L, Korotych O I, Monsalve A G, Wable D, Savliwala S, Grooms N W, Nacea C, Tuitt O R and Dobson J 2019 Evaluation of magnetic nanoparticles for magnetic fluid hyperthermia *Int. J. Hyperth.* **36** 686–700

[116] Montazersaheb P, Pishgahzadeh E, Jahani V B, Farahzadi R and Montazersaheb S 2023 Magnetic nanoparticle-based hyperthermia: a prospect in cancer stem cell tracking and therapy *Life Sci.* **323** 121714

[117] Hu R, Ma S, Li H, Ke X, Wang G, Wei D and Wang W 2011 Effect of magnetic fluid hyperthermia on lung cancer nodules in a murine model *Oncol. Lett.* **2** 1161–4

[118] Shetake N G, Kumar A, Gaikwad S, Ray P, Desai S, Ningthoujam R S, Vatsa R K and Pandey B N 2015 Magnetic nanoparticle-mediated hyperthermia therapy induces tumour growth inhibition by apoptosis and Hsp90/AKT modulation *Int. J. Hyperth.* **31** 909–19

[119] Ryu J, Lee K, Joe C, Joo J, Lee N and Yoo H-S 2018 Patient with unresectable cholangiocarcinoma treated with radiofrequency hyperthermia in combination with chemotherapy: a case report *Integr. Cancer Therap.* **17** 558–61

[120] Belyanina I, Kolovskaya O, Zamay S, Gargaun A, Zamay T and Kichkailo A 2017 Targeted magnetic nanotheranostics of cancer *Molecules* **22** 975

[121] Hude I, Sasse S, Engert A and Bröckelmann P J 2017 The emerging role of immune checkpoint inhibition in malignant lymphoma *Haematologica* **102** 30

[122] Jin H, Qian Y, Dai Y, Qiao S, Huang C, Lu L, Luo Q, Chen J and Zhang Z 2016 Magnetic enrichment of dendritic cell vaccine in lymph node with fluorescent-magnetic nanoparticles enhanced cancer immunotherapy *Theranostics* **6** 2000

[123] Sanz-Ortega L, Rojas J M, Marcos A, Portilla Y, Stein J V and Barber D F 2019 T cells loaded with magnetic nanoparticles are retained in peripheral lymph nodes by the application of a magnetic field *J. Nanobiotechnol.* **17** 1–20

[124] Gondan A I B, Ruiz-de-Angulo A, Zabaleta A, Blanco N G, Cobaleda-Siles B M, García-Granda M J, Padro D, Llop J, Arnaiz B and Gato M 2018 Effective cancer immunotherapy in mice by polyIC-imiquimod complexes and engineered magnetic nanoparticles *Biomaterials* **170** 95–115

[125] Chiang C-S, Lin Y-J, Lee R, Lai Y-H, Cheng H-W, Hsieh C-H, Shyu W-C and Chen S-Y 2018 Combination of fucoidan-based magnetic nanoparticles and immunomodulators enhances tumour-localized immunotherapy *Nat. Nanotechnol.* **13** 746–54

[126] Mejías R, Pérez-Yagüe S, Gutiérrez L, Cabrera L I, Spada R, Acedo P, Serna C J, Lázaro F J, Villanueva Á and del P Morales M 2011 Dimercaptosuccinic acid-coated magnetite nanoparticles for magnetically guided *in vivo* delivery of interferon gamma for cancer immunotherapy *Biomaterials* **32** 2938–52

[127] Jiang H, Fu H, Guo Y, Hu P and Shi J 2022 Evoking tumor associated macrophages by mitochondria-targeted magnetothermal immunogenic cell death for cancer immunotherapy *Biomaterials* **289** 121799

[128] Malumbres A, Martínez G, Mallada R, Hueso J, Bomatí-Miguel O and Santamaría J 2013 Continuous production of iron-based nanocrystals by laser pyrolysis. effect of operating variables on size, composition and magnetic response *Nanotechnology* **24** 325603

[129] Kang J, Kim Y, Kim H-m, Hu X, Saito N, Choi J-H and Lee M-H 2016 In-situ one-step synthesis of carbon-encapsulated naked magnetic metal nanoparticles conducted without additional reductants and agents *Sci. Rep.* **6** 38652

[130] Eremin A, Gurentsov E, Mikheyeva E Y and Musikhin S 2016 Binary iron–carbon nanoparticle synthesis in photolysis of $FeCO_5$ with methane and acetylene *J. Phys.: Conf. Ser.* **774** 012127

[131] Chen M, Gerges M, Raynor W Y, Park P S U, Nguyen E, Chan D H and Gholamrezanezhad A 2024 State of the art imaging of osteoporosis *Semin. Nucl. Med.* **54** 415–26

[132] Farinha P, Coelho J M, Reis C P and Gaspar M M 2021 A comprehensive updated review on magnetic nanoparticles in diagnostics *Nanomaterials* **11** 3432

[133] Sharma K and Chauhan C 2023 Role of magnetic nanoparticle (MNPs) in cancer treatment: a review *Mater. Today Proc.* **81** 919–25

[134] Power S P, Moloney F, Twomey M, James K, O'Connor O J and Maher M M 2016 Computed tomography and patient risk: facts, perceptions and uncertainties *World J. Radiol.* **8** 902

[135] Wei L, Li S, Yang J, Ye Y, Zou J, Wang L, Long R, Zurkiya O, Zhao T and Johnson J 2011 Protein-based MRI contrast agents for molecular imaging of prostate cancer *Mol. Imag. Biol.* **13** 416–23

[136] Mao Y, Li Y, Zang F, Yu H, Yan S, Song Q, Qin Z, Sun J, Chen B and Huang X 2022 Continuous synthesis of extremely small-sized iron oxide nanoparticles used for T1-weighted magnetic resonance imaging via a fluidic reactor *Sci. China Mater.* **65** 1646–54

[137] Kim D, Yu M K, Lee T S, Park J J, Jeong Y Y and Jon S 2011 Amphiphilic polymer-coated hybrid nanoparticles as CT/MRI dual contrast agents *Nanotechnology* **22** 155101

[138] Schwenck J, Sonanini D, Cotton J M, Rammensee H-G, la Fougère C, Zender L and Pichler B J 2023 Advances in PET imaging of cancer *Nat. Rev. Cancer* **23** 474–90

[139] Hagit A, Soenke B, Johannes B and Shlomo M 2010 Synthesis and characterization of dual modality (CT/MRI) core–shell microparticles for embolization purposes *Biomacromolecules* **11** 1600–7

[140] Li W, Xiao F, Bai X and Xu H 2023 Magnetic nanoparticles for food hazard factors sensing: synthesis, modification and application *Chem. Eng. J.* **465** 142816

[141] Xiang Y, Hu C, Wu G, Xu S and Li Y 2023 Nanomaterial-based microfluidic systems for cancer biomarker detection: recent applications and future perspectives *TrAC, Trends Anal. Chem.* **158** 116835

[142] Li Z, Bao Q, Liu C, Li Y, Yang Y and Liu M 2023 Recent advances in microfluidics-based bioNMR analysis *Lab Chip* **23** 1213–25

[143] Proença C A *et al* 2019 Novel enzyme-free immunomagnetic microfluidic device based on $Co_{0.25}Zn_{0.75}Fe_2O_4$ for cancer biomarker detection *Anal. Chim. Acta* **1071** 59–69

[144] Tiwari H, Rai N, Kajal , Salvi P, Singh S K and Gautam V 2023 *Recent advances in nanomaterials-based targeted drug delivery for preclinical cancer diagnosis and therapeutics Bioengineering* **10** 760

[145] Qureshi A, Tufani A, Corapcioglu G and Niazi J H 2020 CdSe/CdS/ZnS nanocrystals decorated with Fe_3O_4 nanoparticles for point-of-care optomagnetic detection of cancer biomarker in serum *Sens. Actuators* B **321** 128431

[146] Ali A, Shah T, Ullah R, Zhou P, Guo M, Ovais M, Tan Z and Rui Y 2021 Review on recent progress in magnetic nanoparticles: synthesis, characterization, and diverse applications *Front. Chem.* **9** 629054

[147] Sosa-Acosta J R, Iriarte-Mesa C, Ortega G A and Díaz-García A M 2020 DNA–iron oxide nanoparticles conjugates: functional magnetic nanoplatforms in biomedical applications *Surface-modified Nanobiomaterials for Electrochemical and Biomedicine Applications* (Cham: Springer) pp 19–47

[148] Han X, Cao M, Zhou B, Yu C, Liu Y, Peng B, Meng L, Wei J-F, Li L and Huang W 2020 Specifically immobilizing His-tagged allergens to magnetic nanoparticles for fast and quantitative detection of allergen-specific IgE in serum samples *Talanta* **219** 121301

[149] Pires F, Silva J C, Ferreira F C and Portugal C A 2024 Heparinized acellular hydrogels for magnetically induced wound healing applications *ACS Appl. Mater. Interfaces* **16** 9908–24

[150] Vu T T, Zhang A, Wang R, Mathew S, Abeywardana T, Beltran-Lemus M, Ma V, Libby M, Thomas D and Wakefield I 2024 Using single antigen specificity magnetic beads for the isolation of specific antibodies against HLA antigens *HLA* **103** e15490

[151] Kallsten M, Ghorasaini M, Hartmann R, Lehmann F, Bergquist J, Kovac L and Lind S B 2020 Magnetic beads for desalting of monoclonal antibodies and antibody–drug conjugates *Anal. Chem.* **92** 9001–7

[152] Oh S, Jung S H, Seo H, Min M-K, Kim B, Hahn Y K, Kang J H and Choi S 2018 Magnetic activated cell sorting (MACS) pipette tip for immunomagnetic bacteria separation *Sensors Actuators* B **272** 324–30

[153] González-Ravina C, Pachec. Castro A, Cru. Palomino M and Requen. Miranda A 2021 P–081 Microfluidic sorting does not improve clinical outcomes compared to magnetic activated cell sorting (MACS) in assisted reproduction *Hum. Reprod.* **36** deab130. 080

[154] Wang L, Lin H, Zhang J and Wang J 2022 Phage long tail fiber protein-immobilized magnetic nanoparticles for rapid and ultrasensitive detection of Salmonella *Talanta* **248** 123627

[155] Lin Z, Lin S-Y, Xie P, Lin C-Y, Rather G M, Bertino J R and Javanmard M 2020 Rapid assessment of surface markers on cancer cells using immuno-magnetic separation and multi-frequency impedance cytometry for targeted therapy *Sci. Rep.* **10** 3015

[156] Wang L, Balasubramanian P, Chen A P, Kummar S, Evrard Y A and Kinders R J 2016 Promise and limits of the CellSearch platform for evaluating pharmacodynamics in circulating tumor cells *Semin. Oncol.* **43** 464–75

[157] Marzougui Z, Chaabouni A, Eissa M M, Elleuch B and Elaissari A 2015 Itaconic acid-functionalized magnetic latex particles for Pb^{2+} removal *Sci. Adv. Mater.* **7** 558–70

[158] Dobson J 2006 Gene therapy progress and prospects: magnetic nanoparticle-based gene delivery *Gene Ther.* **13** 283–7

[159] Kami D, Takeda S, Itakura Y, Gojo S, Watanabe M and Toyoda M 2011 Application of magnetic nanoparticles to gene delivery *Int. J. Mol. Sci.* **12** 3705–22

[160] Vangijzegem T, Stanicki D and Laurent S 2019 Magnetic iron oxide nanoparticles for drug delivery: applications and characteristics *Exp. Opin. Drug Deliv.* **16** 69–78

[161] Xie W, Guo Z, Gao F, Gao Q, Wang D, Liaw B-s, Cai Q, Sun X, Wang X and Zhao L 2018 Shape-, size- and structure-controlled synthesis and biocompatibility of iron oxide nanoparticles for magnetic theranostics *Theranostics* **8** 3284

[162] Keshtkar M, Shahbazi-Gahrouei D and Mahmoudabadi A 2020 Synthesis and application of Fe_3O_4@ Au composite nanoparticles as magnetic resonance/computed tomography dual-modality contrast agent *J. Med. Signals Sens.* **10** 201–7

[163] Gao J, Feng S-S and Guo Y 2010 Antibody Engineering Promotes Nanomedicine for Cancer Treatment *Nanomedicine* **5** 1141–5

[164] Thanh B T, Van Sau N, Ju H, Bashir M J, Jun H K, Phan T B, Ngo Q M, Tran N Q, Hai T H and Van P H 2019 , Immobilization of protein a on monodisperse magnetic nanoparticles for biomedical applications *J. Nanomater.* **2019** 2182471

[165] Bachheti R K, Konwarh R, Gupta V, Husen A and Joshi A 2019 Green synthesis of iron oxide nanoparticles: cutting edge technology and multifaceted applications *Nanomaterials and Plant Potential* (Cham: Springer) pp 239–59

[166] Chen B-W, He Y-C, Sung S-Y, Le T T H, Hsieh C-L, Chen J-Y, Wei Z-H and Yao D-J 2020 Synthesis and characterization of magnetic nanoparticles coated with polystyrene sulfonic acid for biomedical applications *Sci. Technol. Adv. Mater.* **21** 471–81

[167] Bemetz J, Wegemann A, Saatchi K, Haase A, Häfeli U O, Niessner R, Gleich B and Seidel M 2018 Microfluidic-based synthesis of magnetic nanoparticles coupled with miniaturized NMR for online relaxation studies *Anal. Chem.* **90** 9975–82

[168] Ahmed M, Zayed M, El-Dek S, Hady M A, El Sherbiny D H and Uskoković V 2021 Nanofibrous ε-polycaprolactone scaffolds containing Ag-doped magnetite nanoparticles: physicochemical characterization and biological testing for wound dressing applications *in vitro* and *in vivo Bioact. Mater.* **6** 2070–88

[169] Sharma A, Foppen J W, Banerjee A, Sawssen S, Bachhar N, Peddis D and Bandyopadhyay S 2021 Magnetic nanoparticles to unique DNA tracers: effect of functionalization on physico-chemical properties *Nanoscale Res. Lett.* **16** 1–16

[170] Liu T, Chen Z, Li Z, Fu H, Chen G, Feng T and Chen Z 2021 Preparation of magnetic hydrochar derived from iron-rich *Phytolacca acinosa* Roxb. for Cd removal *Sci. Total Environ.* **769** 145159

[171] Dowaidar M, Nasser Abdelhamid H, Hällbrink M, Langel Ü and Zou X 2018 Chitosan enhances gene delivery of oligonucleotide complexes with magnetic nanoparticles–cell-penetrating peptide *J. Biomater. Appl.* **33** 392–401

[172] Zhang F, Li F, Lu G-H, Nie W, Zhang L, Lv Y, Bao W, Gao X, Wei W and Pu K 2019 Engineering magnetosomes for ferroptosis/immunomodulation synergism in cancer *ACS Nano* **13** 5662–73

[173] Fang X, Wang Z, Sun N and Deng C 2021 Magnetic metal oxide affinity chromatography-based molecularly imprinted approach for effective separation of serous and urinary phosphoprotein biomarker *Talanta* **226** 122143

[174] Kusuma K, Manju M, Ravikumar C, Raghavendra N, Kumar T N, Anilkumar M, Nagaswarupa H, Shekhar T S, Murthy H A and Aravind K 2023 Synthesis of strontium oxide nanoparticlesby probe sonication method: its photocatalytic activity and electrochemical sensor studies *Sens. Int.* **4** 100231

[175] Montiel Schneider M G, Martín M J, Otarola J, Vakarelska E, Simeonov V, Lassalle V and Nedyalkova M 2022 Biomedical applications of iron oxide nanoparticles: current insights progress and perspectives *Pharmaceutics* **14** 204

[176] Esquinas-Requena J L, Lozoya-Moreno S, García-Nogueras I, Atienzar-Núñez P, Sánchez-Jurado P M and Abizanda P 2020 La anemia aumenta el riesgo de mortalidad debido a fragilidad *y* discapacidad en mayores: Estudio FRADEA *Aten. Prim.* **52** 452–61

[177] Liu R, Liu X, Lin W and Liu Y 2024 Solvothermal treatment of micron-sized commercial $SrAl_2O_4$: Eu^{2+}, Dy^{3+} phosphors and one-step preparation of nanophosphors for fingerprint imaging *Appl. Sci.* **14** 3929

[178] Liang Y, Jiang L, Xu S, Ju W, Tao Z, Yang Y, Peng X and Wei G 2024 Synthesis and characterization of Fe_3O_4 nanoparticles prepared by solvothermal method *J. Mater. Eng. Perform.* **33** 6804–15

[179] Silva M G D, Santiago L E P, Fernandes R D S, Padilha C E D A and Souza D F D S 2024 Analysis of thermal decomposition of magnetic nanoparticles synthesized by reverse coprecipitation and partial oxidation of ferrous ions *Braz. J. Chem. Eng.* **41** 347–57

[180] Retizlaf A, de Souza Sikora M, Ivashita F F, Schneider R, Botteselle G V and Junior H E Z 2023 $CoFe_2O_4$ magnetic nanoparticles: synthesis by thermal decomposition of 8-hydroxyquinolinates, characterization, and application in catalysis *MRS Commun.* **13** 567–73

[181] Fathi A, Ahmadi M, Madrakian T, Afkhami A and Asadi S 2023 A multi-nebulizer-based aerosol-assisted system for the synthesis of magnetic iron mixed metal oxides nanoparticles (MFe_2O_4, M = Fe^{2+}, Ni^{2+}, Mn^{2+}, Co^{2+}, Zn^{2+}) *Chem. Pap.* **77** 6933–46

[182] Jia F, Zhou S, Liu J, Du J, Dong W, Xue W, Chen L, Yang Y, Wei Y and Yu S 2024 Metal-modified carbon dots: synthesis, properties, and applications in cancer diagnosis and treatment *Appl. Mater. Today* **37** 102133

[183] Bentarhlia N, Elansary M, Belaiche M, Mouhib Y, Lemine O, Zaher H, Oubihi A, Kartah B and Monfalouti H 2023 Evaluating of novel Mn–Mg–Co ferrite nanoparticles for biomedical applications: from synthesis to biological activities *Ceram. Int.* **49** 40421–34

[184] Yashpreet Y and Chudasama B 2023 Magnetic hyperthermia of polyvinylpyrrolidone coated $La_{0.6}Sr_{0.4}MnO_3$ nanoparticles synthesized by sol–gel auto combust method *J. Nano Res.* **77** 27–46

[185] Fopase R, Pandey L M, Hazarika K P, Borah J P, Singh R K and Srinivasan A 2024 Enhancement in the induction heating efficacy of sol–gel derived SiO_2–CaO–Na_2O–P_2O_5 bioglass-ceramics by incorporating magnetite nanoparticles *J. Mater. Chem.* B **12** 3494–508

[186] Alkhalidi H M, Zaman U, Khan D, ur Rehman K, Omar K I, Alissa M, Rizg W Y, Bukhary D M, Abdelrahman E A and Refat M S 2023 Microwave assisted eco-benign synthesis of novel palladium nanoparticles (ACPs-PdNPs): a new insight into photocatalytic and biomedical applications *J. Mol. Liq.* **392** 123469

[187] Chircov C, Bîrcă A C, Dănciulescu L A, Neacşu I A, Oprea O-C, Truşcă R-D and Andronescu E 2023 Usnic acid-loaded magnetite nanoparticles—a comparative study between synthesis methods *Molecules* **28** 5198

[188] Singh V P, Singh C P, Ranjan H and Pandey S K 2024 Synthesis and characterization of iron oxide nanoparticles for bio-medical and neuromorphic computing applications *2024 Int. Conf. on Smart Grid and Energy (ICSGE)* (Piscataway, NJ: IEEE) pp 38–42

[189] Dwivedi A, Das S, Tiwari V, Yadav V, Jain S K, Mandal V, Mukherjee S, Satpathy S, Mohapatra D and Sahu A N 2024 Microwave-assisted green synthesis of silver nanoparticles using *Mitragyna parvifolia* bark extract and their biological activities: an economical and environment-friendly approach *Green Chem. Lett. Rev.* **17** 2395919

[190] Minbashi M, Kordbacheh A A, Ghobadi A and Tuchin V V 2020 Optimization of power used in liver cancer microwave therapy by injection of magnetic nanoparticles (MNPs) *Comput. Biol. Med.* **120** 103741

[191] Salvador M, Gutiérrez G, Noriega S, Moyano A, Blanco-López M C and Matos M 2021 Microemulsion synthesis of superparamagnetic nanoparticles for bioapplications *Int. J. Mol. Sci.* **22** 427

[192] Asab G, Zereffa E A and Abdo Seghne T 2020 Synthesis of silica-coated Fe_3O_4 nanoparticles by microemulsion method: characterization and evaluation of antimicrobial activity *Int. J. Biomater.* **2020** 4783612

[193] Carrillo-Gaytan R P, Rivera-Rangel R D, Razo-Lazcano T A, Falcón-Millán G and González-Muñoz M P 2024 Synthesis of AuNPs in microemulsion and nano-emulsion systems using aqueous extract of *C. chayamansa* leaves as reducing agent *Colloids Surf.*, A **687** 133460

[194] Kaur T and Sharma D 2024 Self-propelling bacteria-based magnetic nanoparticles (BacMags) for targeted magnetic hyperthermia therapy against hypoxic tumors *Nanoscale* **16** 7892–907

[195] Satarzadeh N, Shakibaie M, Forootanfar H and Amirheidari B 2024 Purification, characterization, and assessment of anticancer activity of iron oxide nanoparticles biosynthesized by novel thermophilic *Bacillus tequilensis* ASFS1 *J. Basic Microbiol.* **64** e2400153

[196] Rehman S, Almessiere M A, A. Al-Suhaimi E, Hussain M, Yousuf Bari M, Mehmood Ali S, Al-Jameel S S, Slimani Y, Khan F A and Baykal A 2021 Ultrasonic synthesis and biomedical application of $Mn_{0.5}Zn_{0.5}Er_xY_xFe_{2-2x}O_4$ nanoparticles *Biomolecules* **11** 703

[197] Vicente T T, Arsalani S, Quiel M S, Fernandes G S, da Silva K R, Fukada S Y, Gualdi A J, Guidelli É J, Baffa O and Carneiro A A 2024 Improving the theranostic potential of magnetic nanoparticles by coating with natural rubber latex for ultrasound, photoacoustic imaging, and magnetic hyperthermia: an *in vitro* study *Pharmaceutics* **16** 1474

[198] Patel H, Upadhyay R, Parekh K, Reis D, Oliveira C L and Neto A F 2024 Optimized $Mn_{0.5}Zn_{0.5}Fe_2O_4$ nanoflowers based magnetic fluids for potential biomedical applications *J. Magn. Magn. Mater.* **590** 171656

[199] Chen R, Canales A and Anikeeva P 2017 Neural recording and modulation technologies *Nat. Rev. Mater.* **2** 1–16

[200] Thomas G, Boudon J, Maurizi L, Moreau M, Walker P, Severin I, Oudot A, Goze C, Poty S and Vrigneaud J-M 2019 Innovative magnetic nanoparticles for PET/MRI bimodal imaging *ACS Omega* **4** 2637–48

[201] Ovejero J G, Spizzo F, Morales M P and Del Bianco L 2021 Nanoparticles for magnetic heating: when two (or more) is better than one *Materials* **14** 6416

[202] Van de Walle A, Perez J E, Abou-Hassan A, Hémadi M, Luciani N and Wilhelm C 2020 Magnetic nanoparticles in regenerative medicine: what of their fate and impact in stem cells? *Mater. Today Nano* **11** 100084

[203] Lavorato G C, Das R, Xing Y, Robles J, Litterst F J, Baggio-Saitovitch E, Phan M-H and Srikanth H 2020 , Origin and shell-driven optimization of the heating power in core/shell bimagnetic nanoparticles *ACS Appl. Nano Mater.* **3** 1755–65
[204] Fabris F, Lima E, De Biasi E, Troiani H E, Mansilla M V, Torres T E, Pacheco R F, Ibarra M R, Goya G F and Zysler R D 2019 Controlling the dominant magnetic relaxation mechanisms for magnetic hyperthermia in bimagnetic core–shell nanoparticles *Nanoscale* **11** 3164–72
[205] Yang F, Skripka A, Benayas A, Dong X, Hong S H, Ren F, Oh J K, Liu X, Vetrone F and Ma D 2018 An integrated multifunctional nanoplatform for deep-tissue dual-mode imaging *Adv. Funct. Mater.* **28** 1706235
[206] Kim M R, Xu Z, Chen G and Ma D 2014 Semiconductor and metallic core–shell nanostructures: synthesis and applications in solar cells and catalysis *Chem. Eur. J.* **20** 11256–75
[207] Ma D 2019 Hybrid nanoparticles: an introduction *Noble Metal–Metal Oxide Hybrid Nanoparticles* (Amsterdam: Elsevier) pp 3–6
[208] Atwater H A and Polman A 2010 Plasmonics for improved photovoltaic devices *Nat. Mater.* **9** 205–13
[209] Parameswaran Sreekala A 2023 Hybrid Nanomaterials for Photodetectors with Extended Wavelength Range and High Efficiency *PhD* Universidad Autónoma de Nuevo León http://eprints.uanl.mx/id/eprint/25751
[210] Song G, Kenney M, Chen Y-S, Zheng X, Deng Y, Chen Z, Wang S X, Gambhir S S, Dai H and Rao J 2020 Carbon-coated FeCo nanoparticles as sensitive magnetic-particle-imaging tracers with photothermal and magnetothermal properties *Nat. Biomed. Eng.* **4** 325–34
[211] He S, Zhang H, Liu Y, Sun F, Yu X, Li X, Zhang L, Wang L, Mao K and Wang G 2018 Maximizing specific loss power for magnetic hyperthermia by hard–soft mixed ferrites *Small* **14** 1800135
[212] Wu L, Mendoza-Garcia A, Li Q and Sun S 2016 Organic phase syntheses of magnetic nanoparticles and their applications *Chem. Rev.* **116** 10473–512
[213] Nandwana V, Zhou R, Mohapatra J, Kim S, Prasad P V, Liu J and Dravid V P 2018 Exchange coupling in soft magnetic nanostructures and its direct effect on their theranostic properties *ACS Appl. Mater. Interfaces* **10** 27233–43
[214] Wang L, Yan Y, Wang M, Yang H, Zhou Z, Peng C and Yang S 2016 An integrated nanoplatform for theranostics via multifunctional core–shell ferrite nanocubes *J. Mater. Chem.* B **4** 1908–14
[215] Jiang G, Huang Y, Zhang S, Zhu H, Wu Z and Sun S 2016 Controlled synthesis of Au–Fe heterodimer nanoparticles and their conversion into Au–Fe_3O_4 heterostructured nanoparticles *Nanoscale* **8** 17947–52
[216] Das R, Rinaldi-Montes N, Alonso J, Amghouz Z, Garaio E, Garcia J A, Gorria P, Blanco J A, Phan M-H and Srikanth H 2016 Boosted hyperthermia therapy by combined AC magnetic and photothermal exposures in Ag/Fe_3O_4 nanoflowers *ACS Appl. Mater. Interfaces* **8** 25162–9
[217] Curcio A, Silva A K, Cabana S, Espinosa A, Baptiste B, Menguy N, Wilhelm C and Abou-Hassan A 2019 Iron oxide nanoflowers@ CuS hybrids for cancer tri-therapy: interplay of photothermal therapy, magnetic hyperthermia and photodynamic therapy *Theranostics* **9** 1288
[218] Nicolás-Boluda A, Vaquero J, Laurent G, Renault G, Bazzi R, Donnadieu E, Roux S, Fouassier L and Gazeau F 2020 Photothermal depletion of cancer-associated fibroblasts normalizes tumor stiffness in desmoplastic cholangiocarcinoma *ACS Nano* **14** 5738–53

[219] Bordet A, Landis R F, Lee Y, Tonga G Y, Asensio J M, Li C-H, Fazzini P-F, Soulantica K, Rotello V M and Chaudret B 2019 Water-dispersible and biocompatible iron carbide nanoparticles with high specific absorption rate *ACS Nano* **13** 2870–8
[220] Dong J and Zink J I 2014 Taking the temperature of the interiors of magnetically heated nanoparticles *ACS Nano* **8** 5199–207
[221] Noh S-h, Na W, Jang J-t, Lee J-H, Lee E J, Moon S H, Lim Y, Shin J-S and Cheon J 2012 Nanoscale magnetism control via surface and exchange anisotropy for optimized ferrimagnetic hysteresis *Nano Lett.* **12** 3716–21
[222] Jiang L and Li X 2024 Synthesis and characterisation of PEG-coated $CoFe_2O_4$-based nanoparticles as anticancer nano-delivery systems *Mater. Lett.* **372** 137013
[223] Zhou Z, Zhou H, Zhang K, Wang Y, Gao Y, Liu F, Yang H and Yang S 2021 ZnDPA-conjugated cyanine probes for targeted near-infrared fluorescence and photoacoustic imaging of drug-induced liver injury *in vivo Dyes Pigm.* **194** 109586
[224] Kandasamy G and Maity D 2021 Multifunctional theranostic nanoparticles for biomedical cancer treatments—a comprehensive review *Mater. Sci. Eng.* C **127** 112199
[225] Cazares-Cortes E, Wilhelm C, Perez J E, Espinosa A, Casale S, Michel A, Abou-Hassan A and Ménager C 2021 Tuning the load of gold and magnetic nanoparticles in nanogels through their design for enhanced dual magneto-photo-thermia *Chem. Commun.* **57** 5945–8
[226] Kulpa-Greszta M, Tomaszewska A, Dziedzic A, Rzeszutek I and Pązik R 2023 Heat generation on Fe_3O_4@ SiO_2@ Au core–shell structures using the synergy of an alternating magnetic field and NIR laser light within Ist biological optical window *Mater. Today Commun.* **35** 105513
[227] Chen Y, Xu C, Cheng Y and Cheng Q 2021 Photostability enhancement of silica-coated gold nanostars for photoacoustic imaging guided photothermal therapy *Photoacoustics* **23** 100284
[228] Shams S F, Ghazanfari M R, Pettinger S, Tavabi A H, Siemensmeyer K, Smekhova A, Dunin-Borkowski R E, Westmeyer G G and Schmitz-Antoniak C 2020 Structural perspective on revealing heat dissipation behavior of $CoFe_2O_4$–Pd nanohybrids: great promise for magnetic fluid hyperthermia *Phys. Chem. Chem. Phys.* **22** 26728–41
[229] Keyvan Rad J, Alinejad Z, Khoei S and Mahdavian A R 2019 Controlled release and photothermal behavior of multipurpose nanocomposite particles containing encapsulated gold-decorated magnetite and 5-FU in poly (lactide-co-glycolide) *ACS Biomater. Sci. Eng.* **5** 4425–34
[230] Fan Z, Shelton M, Singh A K, Senapati D, Khan S A and Ray P C 2012 Multifunctional plasmonic shell–magnetic core nanoparticles for targeted diagnostics, isolation, and photothermal destruction of tumor cells *ACS Nano* **6** 1065–73
[231] Lu Q, Dai X, Zhang P, Tan X, Zhong Y, Yao C, Song M, Song G, Zhang Z and Peng G 2018 Fe_3O_4@ Au composite magnetic nanoparticles modified with cetuximab for targeted magneto-photothermal therapy of glioma cells *Int. J. Nanomed.* **2018** 2491–505
[232] Gandia D, Gandarias L, Marcano L, Orue I, Gil-Cartón D, Alonso J, García-Arribas A, Muela A and Fdez-Gubieda M L 2020 Elucidating the role of shape anisotropy in faceted magnetic nanoparticles using biogenic magnetosomes as a model *Nanoscale* **12** 16081–90
[233] Barati E and Cinal M 2017 Gilbert damping in binary magnetic multilayers *Phys. Rev.* B **95** 134440

Sudip Mukherjee, Vijay Sagar Madamsetty, Lipi Pradhan, Anjali Upadhyay and Devyani Yenurkar

Chapter 3

Magnetic nanoparticles for cancer therapy

Magnetic nanoparticles (MNPs) are promising tools in cancer diagnostics and therapeutics, offering multifunctional solutions. Their superparamagnetic properties enable precise control and enhance imaging techniques like magnetic resonance imaging (MRI), providing high-resolution tumor detection and monitoring. In therapeutics, MNPs are used for magnetic hyperthermia, generating localized heat to selectively destroy cancer cells. They also serve as nanocarriers for targeted drug delivery, ensuring precise therapeutic agent release at tumor sites while minimizing systemic toxicity. When functionalized with biomolecules, MNPs achieve high specificity and biocompatibility. These properties position MNPs as transformative agents for advancing cancer detection, treatment, and personalized medicine.

MNPs are gaining prominence in cancer therapy due to their unique magnetic properties, biocompatibility, and versatility. These nanoparticles are increasingly used in cancer therapy because they can be engineered to carry drugs precisely to tumors, offering more precise and minimally invasive cancer treatment solutions [1]. Because of their small size, MNPs can readily circulate throughout the body and concentrate at tumor sites, particularly when directed by an external magnetic field. MNPs play key roles in several cancer treatment strategies, including roles as drug delivery vehicles and anticancer agents [2]. Their use is not only limited to therapy; MNPs have attracted a lot of interest for their applications in cancer theranostics [1]. MNPs have gained increasing popularity in cancer theranostics due to their distinctive physicochemical features. These include easy surface modification, good biodegradability, easy synthesis, low toxicity, and the ability to enhance MRI contrast [3]. MNPs are widely used in cancer theranostics, including drug delivery, MRI imaging, photodynamic therapy (PDT), biosensors, immunotherapy, radiotherapy, magnetic hyperthermia, and photothermal therapy (PTT), as shown in scheme 3.1 [4].

doi:10.1088/978-0-7503-6335-8ch3

© IOP Publishing Ltd 2025. All rights, including for text and data mining (TDM), artificial intelligence (AI) training, and similar technologies, are reserved.

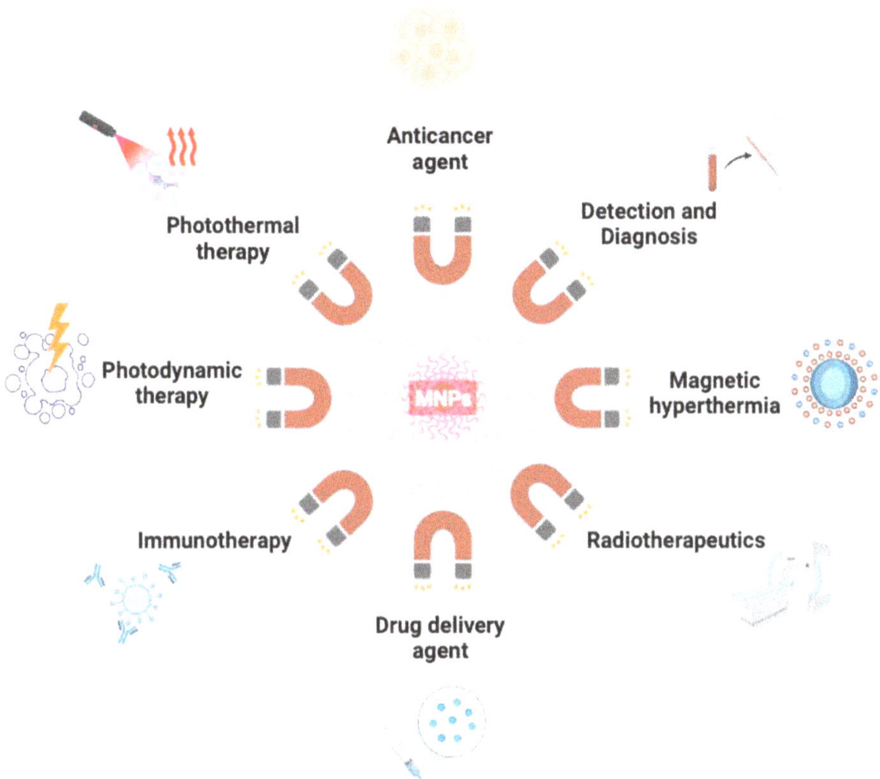

Scheme 3.1. Illustration representing the diversity of MNPs in cancer theranostics.

3.1 MNPs as drug delivery vehicles

As drug delivery vehicles, MNPs are transforming cancer therapy by enhancing the effectiveness of therapy control and targeting. Minimizing collateral adverse effects on healthy tissue is one of the key objectives of cancer treatment research, and this strategy is helping to achieve this end goal [5]. The nanoparticles can be targeted precisely to the tumor location, reducing systemic exposure [6]. Because of this control, MNPs are particularly useful for treating tumors that are surrounded by sensitive tissues or are hard to reach. This leads to the creation of MNP-based drug delivery systems (MDDSs), which often use iron oxide (Fe_2O_3, Fe_3O_4, etc.) as a building block. Additionally, to provide efficient control and delivery of drugs to the desired location, their surface can be functionalized by organic or inorganic modifications [7]. Compared to other drug delivery systems, MDDSs possess potent targeting ability and low side-effect rates. Hence, due to their responsive sensitivity to external magnetic fields, they are considered novel drug delivery systems [8]. In drug delivery, MNPs are collectively used for targeted therapy, controlled drug release, and increasing drug-loading stability and capacity. For instance, retrievable

MNPs for drug delivery using a bilayer hydrogel sheet-type intraocular microrobot were reported by Kim *et al.* They designed MNP retrieval by considering the traditional adverse effects of microrobot saturation in the eye. They reported that an MNP layer and a therapeutic layer made up the bilayer hydrogel microrobot. Applying an alternating magnetic field (AMF) at the target location degraded the therapeutic layer, releasing drug particles, and the MNP layer was subsequently recovered using an AMF. They performed *in vitro* and *ex vivo* studies using retinoblastoma Y79 cancer cells, showing migration of the treatment. Hence, they concluded that MNPs were newer and better alternatives to the existing traditional microrobots for drug delivery [9]. Similarly, drug delivery using retrievable micro-robots was reported by Lee *et al.* They described the use of doxorubicin (DOX), an anticancer drug encapsulated in a biocompatible and hydrolyzable polyethylene glycol diacrylate (PEGDA)-based helical microrobot that could retrieve MNPs, as shown in figure 3.1. In their study, DOX was conjugated to MNPs via a disulfide link. Following precise delivery to the cancer cells via magnetic field alteration, the microrobot offered quick MNP separation. This was possible due to the use of near-infrared (NIR) light as an external stimulus and a reducing agent, dithiothreitol (DTT), which was similar to the surrounding cancer cells. They conducted *in vitro* testing using the liver cancer cell line Huh-7. They confirmed the release of the drug from this delivery system and treated the cancer cells by successfully separating the MNPs through an external magnetic field [10]. For aggressive cancers such as pancreatic ductal adenocarcinoma, Han and Hou *et al* described a sequential drug delivery strategy based on two steps. Drugs such as metformin were used to enhance

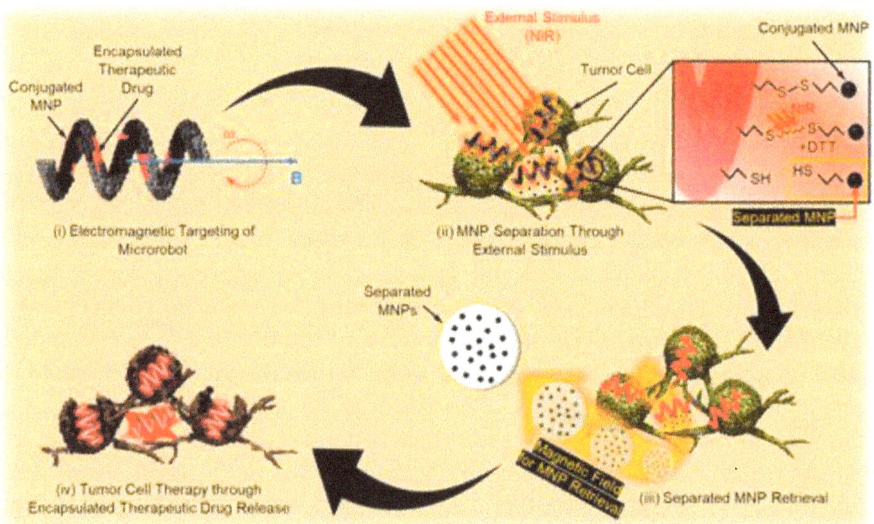

Figure 3.1. Concept of the MNP-based retrievable helical-type microrobot, showing the process of active electromagnetic targeting, NIR irradiation for external stimulus, MNP separation after weakening the conjugation between the helical-type structure and the MNPs, and separated MNP retrieval using a dynamic magnetic field. Adapted with permission from [10]. Copyright (2021) American Chemical Society.

the penetration of gemcitabine present in the MNPs. The researchers described a mechanism in which metformin inhibited the generation of the fibrogenic cytokine TGF-β3, resulting in the reduction of pancreatic stellate cells (PSCs) by the adenosine monophosphate-activated protein kinase pathway of tumor cells. *In vivo*, orthotopic and subcutaneous mouse models demonstrated a reduction of 91.2% in tumor growth after 30 days of treatment. Therefore, this study showed that this type of targeted cancer therapy based on a two-step mechanism improves efficiency [11]. In another study, MNPs were encapsulated to deliver the extract of pomegranate peel, which was further coated with chitosan for the treatment of breast cancer. This delivery by MNPs showed 60% scavenging activity in an antioxidant assay and was confirmed to be nontoxic to normal cells [12]. Similarly, another study by Dhavale *et al* used chitosan-coated MNPs for the delivery of the anticancer drug telmisartan. They enhanced the therapeutic activity of telmisartan, a drug that is poorly soluble; hence, the MNPs helped to increase the drug loading due to the larger surface area provided by the chitosan coating. This stable formulation released the drug efficiently in the tumor environment. *In vitro* studies were conducted using PC-3 human prostate cancer cells, demonstrating cytotoxicity against cancer cells [13]. In an ovarian cancer study, multifunctional nanoparticles coupled with methotrexate were designed using chitosan to deliver erlotinib. The polymerizable organo-soluble precursor was created by modifying chitosan with maleic anhydride and sodium dodecyl sulfate. Furthermore, chitosan was functionalized by free radical polymerization using pH- and temperature-sensitive monomers. Following that, a complex between the carboxylic acid groups of the synthesized chitosan copolymer MNPs was developed by Fathi *et al.* The average size of this complex was 112 nm, with a charge of −28.4 mV. They reported a loading efficiency of 17% of MNPs to 86% of erlotinib. The NPs with erlotinib carried out both pH- and thermal-based drug delivery, whereas NPs loaded with both erlotinib and methotrexate were found to be toxic to the OVCAR-3 cell line. They concluded that the nanocomplex proved to be an effective alternative for targeted cancer therapy [14]. For example, the MNPs were synthesized using a coprecipitation method with a narrow size distribution, and their surface was modified with biocompatible materials such as polyvinyl alcohol (PVA) and layered double hydroxides (LDHs) to enhance stability, reduce toxicity, and improve biocompatibility. A thermal analysis indicated that the coated nanoparticles had higher thermal stability than uncoated ones. However, an evaluation of their magnetic properties showed that they were depleted, which was attributed to the effect of surface modification. This study highlighted the effectiveness of the coated MNPs in drug delivery, showing improved drug release kinetics and enhanced potency against HepG2 liver cancer cells without cytotoxicity toward normal fibroblast cells (3T3). Additionally, a magnetic evaluation confirmed that the surface modification preserved the superparamagnetic behavior of the MNPs, which is crucial for their functionality in targeted drug delivery systems [15]. In another study, magnetic mesoporous NPs were designed to provide magnetic properties and were coated with mesoporous silica that allowed for effective drug loading and controlled release. This study reported that folic acid (FA) functionalized these MNPs, enhancing their targeting ability toward cancer cells that overexpress folate receptors, such as HeLa cells. They demonstrated a significant increase in cytotoxicity *in vitro* against HeLa cells compared to non-targeted formulations, indicating the effectiveness of folate-receptor-mediated endocytosis in drug delivery. The release profile of the anticancer drug from these MNPs was evaluated at different pH levels, revealing a higher release rate at acidic pH values compared to neutral pH values, which is beneficial when targeting tumor environments [16].

3.2 MNPs as anticancer agents

Cancer therapy failure is generally caused by drug resistance [17]. Cancer targeting can be maximized by these novel drug delivery systems based on nanoparticles, which offer sustained drug release, effective tissue penetration, increased absorption by cancer cells, and better organelle-targeted delivery [18]. In a study, MNPs were tested using HeLa cells. The MNPs were synthesized using the coprecipitation method and functionalized using carboxylates. Following this, the drug DOX was used after conjugation with surface modifiers such as citric acid, ascorbic acid, and succinic acid, and thoroughly characterized using dynamic light scattering (DLS) and transmission electron microscopy (TEM), as shown in figure 3.2. The researchers reported the monodisperse formulation of functionalized carboxylates having efficient colloidal stability and magnetic properties. The combination of DOX and carboxylates resulted in higher drug loading due to intermolecular forces. This study compared the drug quantities released by the aforementioned surface-modified MNPs and confirmed that the maximum loading efficiency was achieved through the use of ascorbic acid. However, the succinic-acid-modified MNPs showed less toxicity due to the maximum release of the drug [19]. In another study, MNPs with mesoporous silica-type NPs were designed as a drug delivery system for disulfiram (DSF). Solak *et al* reported the modification of these NPs using polyethylenimine, which was linked with FA (PEI-FA) for better solubility and specificity with tumor cells. High-performance liquid chromatography indicated that this drug system possessed a drug-loading capacity of 4.35%. The optimal drug release kinetics of the drug system were shown to occur at 37 °C and pH 6.0 at the endosome pH level. The researchers stated that these MNPs were captured more frequently by tumor cells than by normal cells under an applied magnetic field. They reported the highest anticancer effect in MCF-7 cells was achieved by a combination consisting of DSF, sodium nitroprusside, and copper ions in an *in vitro* model [20]. Green synthesis based on the active oil of *Satureja hortensis* was used to synthesize MNPs for anticancer, antibacterial, and antifungal purposes. These synthesized NPs were thoroughly characterized using different techniques. The average particle size was 9.3–27 nm, and the particles exhibited cubic crystallography. The researchers reported that the efficiency of the synthesized particles showed enhanced antimicrobial properties compared to the parent essential oil in gram-negative bacteria. Moreover, the antitumor effect was tested *in vitro* using MCF-7 and K-562 cell lines, demonstrating the anticancer effect of these MNPs [21]. In a study of breast cancer, thymoquinone (TQ)-loaded MNPs (TQ-MNPs) were formulated to enhance therapeutic efficiency and bioavailability. Following characterization, the release profile

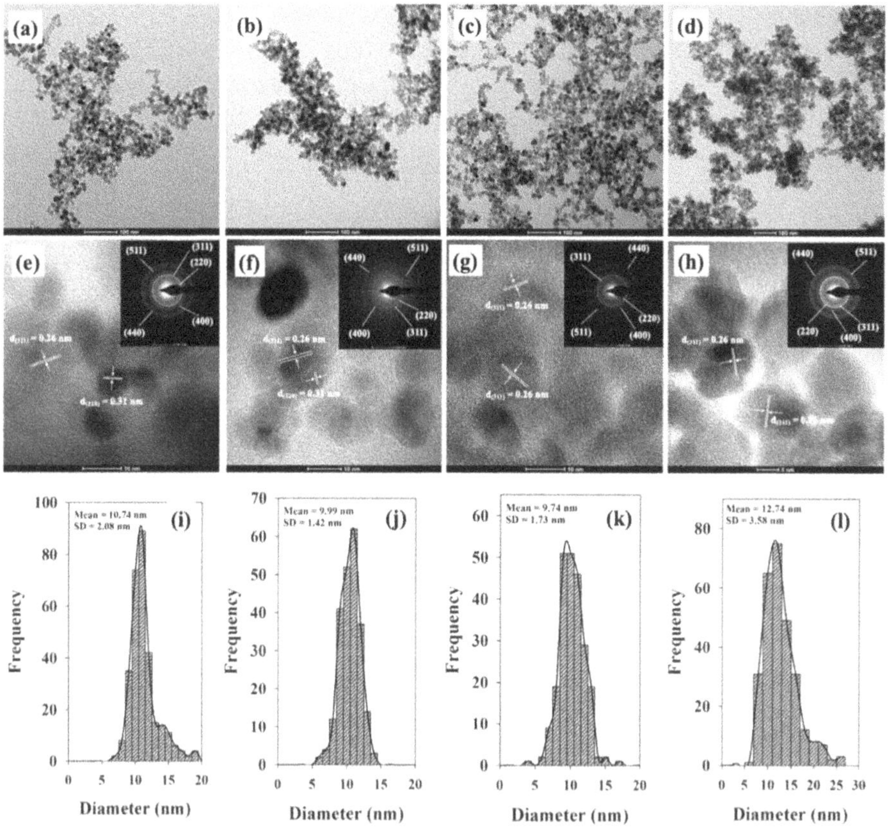

Figure 3.2. (a–d) TEM images, (e–h) high-resolution TEM (HRTEM) images (inset: selected area electron diffraction (SAED)), and (i–l) the corresponding particle size distribution of the as-prepared SA-MNPs, AA-MNPs, CA-MNPs, and unmodified MNPs, respectively. Adapted from [19], Copyright (2020), with permission from Elsevier.

of the MNPs was evaluated to confirm the drug loading by mimicking the delivery environment. According to the investigation, the drug release profile of the TQ-MNPs showed enhanced efficiency. The TQ-MNPs supported anti-proliferation and apoptosis in the breast cancer cell line MCF-7 [22]. Alavi *et al* synthesized chitosan MNPs with iron oxide, which were loaded with atorvastatin for coronal pathogenesis and anti-angiogenesis. An *in vitro* study was carried out using C6 glioma cells; the results suggested that these MNPs inhibited proliferation, induced reactive oxygen species (ROS), and induced apoptotic cell death. In an *in vivo* study using a glioblastoma multiforme mouse model, the researchers reported an increase in the survival rate of the animals due to the reduction in tumor size. The MNPs may upregulate apoptotic proteins such as p53, caspase 3, and Bax, and downregulate anti-apoptotic factors such as vascular endothelial growth factor (VEGF), brain-derived neurotrophic factor (BDNF), and Bcl-2, which are important for tumor development, according to the quantitative reverse transcriptase polymerase chain reaction (qRT-PCR) results [23]. In another study, MNPs were synthesized and characterized for their potential application in cancer therapy, particularly against human ovarian cancer cells. The researchers highlighted the preparation of both PEG-coated and uncoated MNPs using a one-pot hydrothermal method, which resulted in a change in their average sizes. The cytotoxic effects of these MNPs inhibited the proliferation of SKOV-3 ovarian cancer cells, especially when combined with NIR laser irradiation and AMF exposure. This research underscores the potential of MNPs as effective anticancer agents, as no significant adverse effects were observed on liver function enzymes, and no histological alterations took place in spleen and lung tissues [24].

3.3 Immunomodulation and immunotherapy by MNPs

The magnetic characteristics of MNPs make it possible to use magnetic navigation and magnet-based hyperthermia to enhance the impact of immunotherapy [25]. To improve antitumor immune effects, MNPs can utilize selective magnetic hyperthermia to cause immunogenic cell death of tumor cells for efficient antigen release and delivery [26]. Along with this, they can shift tumor-associated macrophages (TAMs) to the M1 phenotype for enhanced tumor-killing capacity [27]. Improved spatiotemporal control over the delivery, release, and dosage of immunomodulatory drugs within the body is one benefit of magnetic systems for enhancing the potency of immunotherapies [28]. This leads to lower off-target effects [29]. A new therapy to treat breast cancer using MNPs to trigger an immune response was reported by Wang *et al.* MNPs can release Fe^{+2} ions for the Fenton reaction, which leads to the production of ROS and hydroxyl free radicals. These are responsible for destroying tumor cells in the presence of weak acidity and excess hydrogen peroxide in the surrounding tumor. The MNPs were responsible for the conversion of M2 to M1 macrophages due to the encouraged maturation of dendritic cells, which resulted in more T cells infiltrating and changing the immunobiology of cancer from a ‘cold’ to a ‘hot’ state. Apart from this, they were also responsible for altering cytokine secretion by tumor cells. Hence, they achieved a synergistic effect by combining imaging with treatment [30]. In another study, a maghemite core consisting of MNPs was synthesized using different coatings (dimercaptosuccinic acid, carboxymethyl dextran, and dextran). These MNPs were evaluated for compatibility with plasma proteins, macrophages, and red blood cells (RBCs). Carboxymethyl dextran-based MNPs (CMD–MNPs) were reported have a better proinflammatory response against macrophages. Hence, micro ribonucleic acid (miRNA) was delivered using the CMD–MNP system. The researchers found that the proinflammatory response due to the upregulation of TNF-α, IL-6, and CD80 was caused by the MNPs in macrophages. Therefore, they suggested a system with miRNA delivery as a novel MNP-based therapeutic tool [31]. A study by Jiang *et al* described a way to detect ferroptosis and induce immunogenicity, which resulted in an increase in the non-inflammatory response to immunotherapy in cancer. They reported biomimetic sulfasalazine (SAS)-loaded MNPs synthesized from platelet membranes. This helped to inhibit the glutamate–cystine antiporter system, resulting in ferroptotic cell death. In an *in vivo* tumor metastasis model, MNPs eliminated the tumor and increased the effectiveness of programmed cell death 1 immune checkpoint inhibitor treatment. According to proteomics research, MNP-mediated ferroptosis has the ability to repolarize macrophages from M2 to M1, promoting an immune response specific to the tumor. Hence, researchers confirmed the potential of ferroptosis-mediated MNPs using the metastasis model [32]. The genetically modified MNPs, which activated immune responses by macrophages, provided immunotherapy, as reported by Rao *et al.* Initially, the cellular uptake of tumor cells by macrophage phagocytosis was inhibited when CD47 bound to a protein present on the macrophage (SIRPα). After this, tumor cells led to the conversion of TAMs into M2 due to the colony-promoting factors. Both of these functions were reversed by the genetically modified MNPs via overexpression of SIRPα, which led to the inhibition of the SIRPα-CD47 pathway. This resulted in the production of strong immune responses by the macrophage. Moreover, the MNPs were directed to the cancer cells with the help of a magnetic field, and the cell membrane coating present on the MNPs provided protection from excretion, contributing to accumulation and circulation. *In vivo* models of breast cancer and melanoma were studied for these modified MNPs, which showed inhibition of metastasis and tumor growth, resulting in extended survival in mice [33]. Similarly, another study presented a dual-pronged chemo–immunotherapy approach that used MNPs coated with mannan and loaded with prodigiosin to repolarize TAM and inhibit the growth of breast tumors. These MNPs had a size of less than 100 nm and exhibited sustained release. Evaluation of the MNPs suggested that they had less cytotoxicity toward normal cells compared to tumor cells. In addition, the MNPs caused an alteration in the dynamics of macrophage polarization in their immunomodulatory activity. This confirmed the targeted application of breast cancer therapy [34]. An *in vivo* model of melanoma and an *in vitro* model of bone marrow-derived macrophages were used to evaluate carboxymethylated β-D-glucan MNPs. These NPs upregulated M1 expression in the macrophage-derived model with a high rate of apoptosis (80.39%), whereas migration was inhibited in the melanoma tumor model. Treatment with MNPs enhanced the CD8 and CD4 lymphocyte infiltration rates in tumors, resulting in cell death [35]. In another study, the use of MNPs was evaluated for the activation and proliferation of natural killer cells in liver cancer. The synthesis of MNPs with the help of DNA was reported, which induced heat and was modified using FA and polyethylenimine [36]. Similarly, Wu *et al* reported the synthesis of MNPs with a coating of SiO_2, forming cell membrane-coated MNPs for the activation of natural killer cells, which were used for anticancer therapy (figure 3.3). The MNPs were modified with antigens specific to tumor cells, activating the killer cells through their overexpression of cytotoxic agents, thereby increasing anticancer activity. This method of coating cancer cell membranes onto MNPs serves as a potential approach for activating killer cells. Thus, the toxicity of natural killer cells is enhanced by increasing the production of cytotoxic agents and using receptors. This was tested *in vitro* using melanoma cells and hepatoma cells, which demonstrated the activation of cells due to the presence of antigens that significantly resulted in cell killing [37].

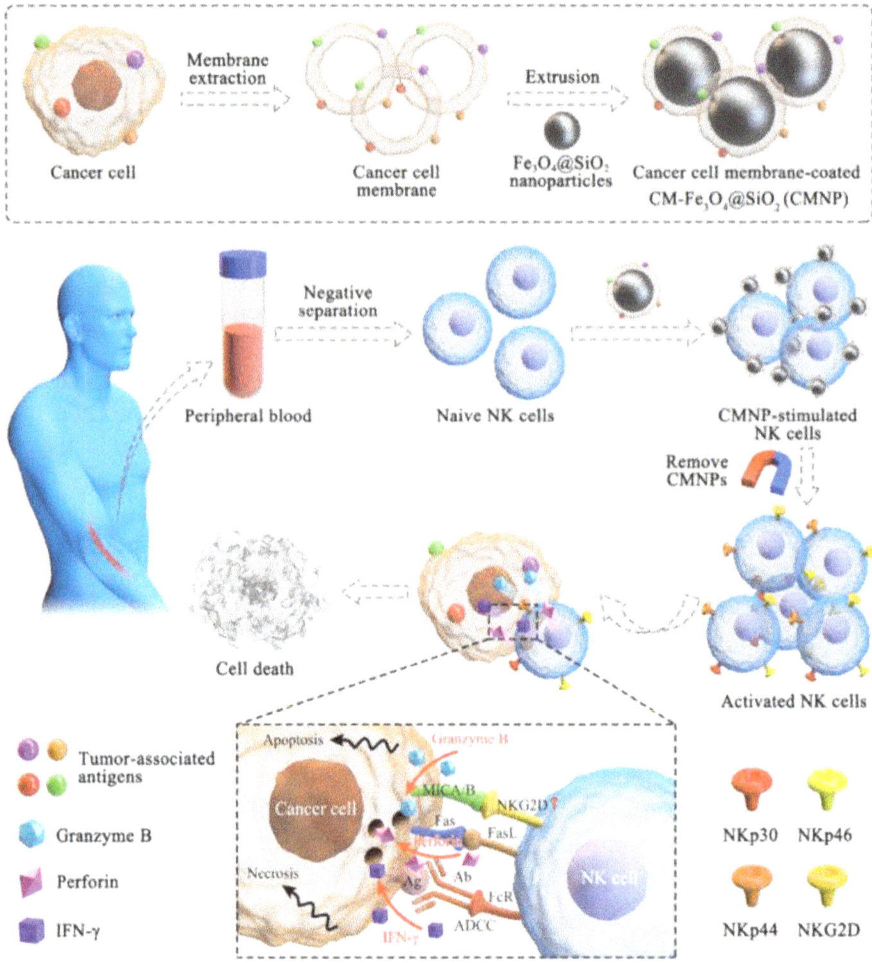

Figure 3.3. Schematic depicting the synthesis of cancer-cell-membrane-coated nanoparticles (CMNPs) and their stimulation of natural killer cells for elevated tumor-killing responses. Adapted from [37], Copyright (2021), with permission from Elsevier.

To enhance the effectiveness of vaccinations, Zn-doped MNPs were created to promote the collaborative activation of immune responses via Toll-like receptor (TLR) signaling. This study highlighted that the combination of TLR agonists with MNPs significantly boosted the immune response against cancer cells, particularly in the context of aggressive B16–F10 melanoma cells expressing the model antigen ovalbumin (OVA). They reported that the MNPs not only enhanced the delivery of these TLR agonists but also allowed for real-time tracking of vaccine migration from the injection site to lymph nodes and tumors using MRI. Moreover, they found that the incorporation of MNPs in the vaccine formulation led to a marked increase in antibodies, indicating a stronger immune response compared to vaccines without MNPs. The researchers concluded that checkpoint inhibition with TLR agonists and

MNPs is important for developing effective cancer immunotherapies [38]. In another study, the development of fucoidan–dextran-based MNPs was designed to deliver checkpoint inhibitors and T cell activators directly to tumors. With magnetic navigation, this system accumulated at the tumor site more efficiently, thereby minimizing off-target effects and enhancing therapeutic outcomes. The results indicated that this therapy reduced side effects, thus increasing the survival rate. The incorporated fucoidan possessed immunomodulating properties that addressed immunosuppression at the tumor site and restored lymphocyte infiltration [39]. This study reported that MNPs can successfully alter immunological responses, particularly when loaded with plant pathogen lipooligosaccharides (LOSs). The addition of MNPs assists in countering the inhibitory immunological pathways that can be triggered when dendritic cells are subjected to TLR4 agonists, resulting in a more positive immune response. The MNPs used in this immunotherapy were nontoxic and caused no reaction with the dendritic cells. The researchers found that TLRs, when exposed to MNPs, influenced cytokine production and cell viability, which affected the immune response. Additionally, this study demonstrated that MNPs can increase programmed death-ligand 1 (PD-L1) expression in dendrites, suggesting a possible synergy with PD-L1 checkpoint inhibitors that could enhance the effectiveness of cancer vaccines. According to the results, when paired with checkpoint inhibition techniques, MNPs can increase the immunogenicity of TLR4 agonists, resulting in more robust antigen-specific cytotoxic T cell responses and better long-term tumor protection [40]. Similarly, spherical MNPs were created through an oil-in-water microemulsion template method by Ge *et al* to improve the traditional limitations of PTT. These MNPs acted as drug vehicles to carry drugs for controlled release. The MNPs were combined with immune checkpoint blockade therapies to enhance the immune response against tumors. In addition to killing tumor cells, PTT ablation stimulates the immune system and helps T cells recognize cancer-associated antigens, increasing the overall effectiveness of treatment. Hence, MNPs combined with immune adjuvants such as R837 and the use of PTT trigger a robust antitumor immune response and prevent metastasis in organs [41]. A study by Grifantini *et al* highlighted that the covalent binding of mAb198.3 to MNPs was unaffected by the conjugation, proving that the antibody's capacity to attach to FAT1-positive colon tumor cells was unaffected. They reported that this system decreased tumor growth *in vivo* at dosages around 200 times lower than the dosage of free mAb198.3, demonstrating the ability of MNPs to enhance the therapeutic effect [42].

3.4 MNP-mediated photothermal therapy

PTT is a thermal-energy-based noninvasive therapy that has attracted interest for use in local cancer treatment. PTT uses an NIR laser to irradiate tumors pretreated with MNPs, creating heat that kills the cancer cells [43]. Longer wavelengths (700–1200 nm) of light can be used for this procedure because they release less energy and cause no harm to nearby healthy tissues [4]. MNPs can produce synergistic effects when combined with other photothermal agents, resulting in greater and more efficient therapeutic effects, making them good candidates for photothermal probes [44]. Their tendency to aggregate overcomes their poor absorption in the NIR region [45]. In the visible and IR spectra, MNPs are reported to exhibit optical absorption due to light-driven activation, which results in localized heating (hyperthermia), making them PTT agents [46]. Li *et al* reported polydopamine-modified MNPs for breast cancer. The polydopamine ensured the potential of these MNPs for use in PTT by enhancing their integrity and durability. The use of these MNPs for PTT removed tumors in 4T1 cell-line-bearing mice. Hence, the researchers described them as an alternative for overcoming the instability and undesirable effects of traditional guided PTT agents [47]. For example, an *in vitro* study was conducted using the MDA-MB-231 cell line, which confirmed that MNPs subjected to light treatment can be taken up by cells, allowing them to act as a probe in imaging. They reported that PTT based on the use of MNPs to achieve heat induction performed better than other methods [48]. In a study, MNPs were used to collect exosomes, and a novel PCR-based photothermal assay was performed to identify the genotype of microRNAs derived from the exosomes. MXenes were inserted into MNPs and used for PTT via NIR control. In this way, temperature-based agarose microcarriers were produced that identified the target with simplicity and precision. A combination of various oncogenes and miRNAs was concurrently and statistically detected in the isolated exosomes using PTT in conjunction with probes. The findings indicated that biomarker levels in normal cells are much lower than in the prostate cancer cell line [49]. PPT was combined with chemotherapy using NPs and nanospheres for the treatment of liver cancer. Compared to NPs, magnetic spheres showed a stronger PTT response. The *in vitro* toxicity of these nanomaterials was evaluated against the HepG2 and THLE-2 cell lines. A dual therapeutic effect was obtained by loading DOX onto the nanomaterials, leading to tumor cell killing. Moreover, this study reported the production of ROS during the treatment, which contributed to a better anticancer effect. These nanomaterials were functionalized and modified with polydopamine. They reduced cell viability because they acted more efficiently under NIR radiation. Thus, this approach toward liver cancer treatment using dendrimer-modified MNPs represents a significant advance in cancer therapy [50]. Similarly, PTT using MNPs was combined with chemotherapy to treat breast cancer. The NPs were synthesized using the hydrothermal method and characterized using various techniques. The 4T1 cell line of breast cancer was used to evaluate the cytotoxicity of MNPs; in addition, biodistribution, cell death, and antitumor activity were investigated. The researchers reported that this combined therapy inhibited tumor growth and effectively delivered the drug at the tumor site without damaging healthy cells. Drug-loaded MNPs in the presence of a magnetic field during PTT, combined with chemotherapy, yielded the maximum effect against tumor cells. Hence, the researchers mentioned that the combination of a magnetic field, chemotherapy, and PTT could be helpful in treating breast cancer [51]. In another study, PTT was used to image glioma cells by loading a photothermal nanoprobe into a macrophage to cross the blood–brain barrier (figure 3.4). This method offered advantages, including MRI, photoacoustic (PA), and fluorescence imaging, for better identification of tumor tissues. The researchers explained that the induction of PTT at the

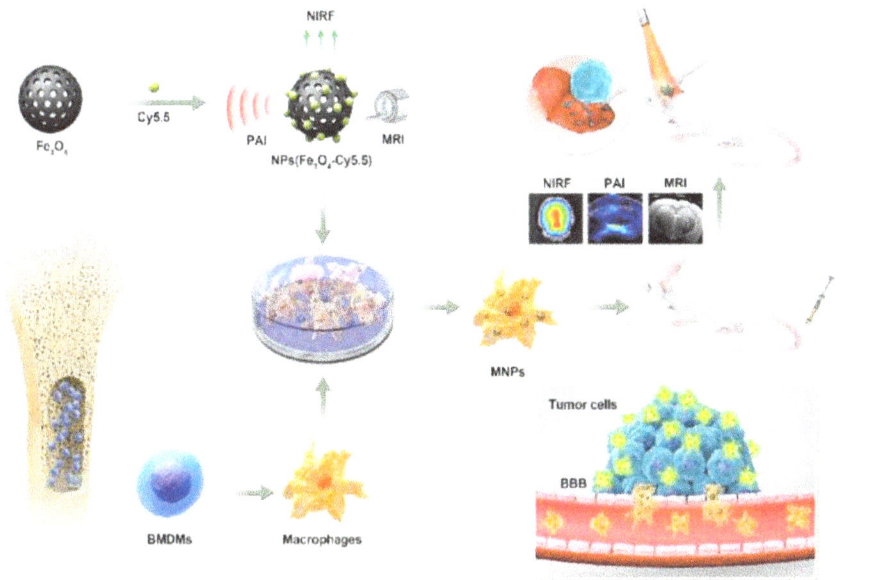

Figure 3.4. Synthetic process and application of MFe_3O_4–Cy5.5[a]. Adapted with permission from [52]. Copyright (2021) American Chemical Society.

local tumor site by the synthesized MNPs resulted in tumor ablation and inhibited the recurrence of the tumor after the resection of the glioma. Hence, this report confirms the importance of the effective action of PTT in diagnostic and therapeutic studies of glioma [52]. An implantable hydrogel incorporating MNPs was used for the PTT of cancer. The MNPs were synthesized by the coprecipitation method to entrap them under an alginate polymer-based implant for the treatment of colon cancer. The CT26 colon cancer cell line was used for this study. Light irradiation incident on cells produced an effective antitumor effect in this treatment [53]. Similarly, a biocompatible polymer was used to modify the MNPs to enhance their internalization by cells and inhibit liver agglomeration and early excretion. In addition, gold particle functionalization was used to enhance the absorption of IR and visible electromagnetic radiation. MNPs with and without the gold coating were compared for PTT, and the results suggested that MNPs with the gold shell coating were more efficient in the visible range. Here, Lazaro *et al* used a dual effect consisting of local hyperthermia carried out by the MNPs and photothermia carried out via PTT [54]. Another study presented a strategy that used membrane-coated MNPs that were hybrids of stem cells from tumors and platelets. These MNPs had superior abilities for immune suppression and targeted treatment. These MNPs utilized special quality platelet membranes, which sent information to avoid immune recognition, and cancer stem cell membranes, which helped with homotypic targeting. The researchers reported that these MNPs were effective in cancer targeting because they increased their uptake by tumor stem cells. *In vivo* studies indicated the highest temperature gain occurred at the tumor site due to laser irradiation, which resulted in effective PTT. In addition to successfully preventing tumor growth, this combination treatment demonstrated improved biological acceptability, as seen by the body weight loss in mice. The effectiveness of the therapy was enhanced by the aggregation of iron in the MNPs at the tumor site for a longer period. Hence, this study highlighted that the strength of the coated MNPs improved immune evasion in the combined therapy [55]. In another study, nano-clusters of MNPs were used to create aggregation near cancer cells due to the magnetic properties produced by the MNPs. These MNPs had inner and outer shells with different functions; the inner shell had a triphenylphosphonium modification on the polydopamine, whereas the outer shell contained methylated PEG, which was separated during a redox reaction and thereby targeted the mitochondria. Magnetic hyperthermia due to laser irradiation damaged the tumor cell membrane, causing cells to undergo apoptosis. This mechanism enhanced therapeutic efficiency by upregulating anticancer drug delivery at the tumor site. As mitochondria of the cell are susceptible to heat, the MNPs, in combination with PTT, proved effective in the treatment of cancer [56]. In a further study, the anticancer drug DOX coated with poly(lactic-co-glycolic) acid (PLGA) was used to create MNPs which were combined with NIR dye. In addition to making magnetic targeting easier, this combination enabled PTT to be used, in which the heat produced by a laser was absorbed by the dye, releasing DOX from the MNPs. Compared to non-targeted methods, the results showed that the application of magnetic targeting increased the concentration of these MNPs in tumors, resulting in improved treatment outcomes. The study showed that when exposed to laser irradiation, the perfluoropentane in the MNPs may speed up drug release, increasing their overall anticancer performance [57]. Small MNPs were designed and reported by Wang *et al* to improve the potential for cancer therapy. This study emphasized the imaging features of MNPs, which fluoresce and can be used in MRI; these features may be utilized for localization and accurate tumor monitoring. The researchers reported that MNPs demonstrate high photothermal conversion efficiency that enables efficient PTT when introduced to NIR light. The efficiency of MNPs in causing tumor cell death by PTT was demonstrated by *in vivo* investigations where mice treated with MNPs under NIR illumination had substantially less cancer growth than control groups. Furthermore, the results of cytotoxicity tests showed that the MNPs had no effect on healthy cells, which makes them a viable option for secure and efficient tumor therapy [58]. A study by Ren *et al* reported that PTT could be enhanced by chemical inhibitors or genetic methods. Cancer inhibition rates increased markedly in *in vivo* trials when MNPs and autophagy inhibitors were combined, suggesting a synergistic impact. According to this study, the suppression of autophagy postponed cancer regrowth and enhanced the anticancer effects, pointing to a possible approach for more robust treatments for cancer. Overall, the study highlighted how MNPs and autophagy interact, offering the possibility for novel combinations that may improve the effectiveness of PTT for cancer [59]. In a study, MNPs were synthesized for bladder cancer treatment. The researchers reported longer circulation of NPs in the blood, resulting in effective therapeutic action due to aggregation at the tumor site. They mentioned that these MNPs act as a contrast agent and help in the imaging of the tumor due to the coordination of iron ions, while their strong absorption in the NIR region facilitates PA imaging and PTT. They demonstrated that the MNPs led to an improvement in light conversion efficiency, which increased the temperature and resulted in cancer cell ablation [60].

3.5 MNPs in photodynamic therapy

PDT has attracted a lot of interest in the field of cancer therapy over the last decade. It is a type of light treatment where drugs or light sensitizers are directed toward the tumor site [1]. These sensitizers are exposed to light of a specific wavelength, creating stressful conditions by producing ROS, which lead to apoptosis in cancer cells [46]. Hence, PDT has emerged as a new alternative to traditional cancer treatments due to its fewer adverse effects, less intrusive behavior, and effective curative capabilities [61]. For instance, researchers used MNPs to create a drug delivery system. This system was created by altering the surfaces of graphene oxide and camptothecin (CPT) and crosslinking them with amino acids. The researchers observed the pH-dependent release of CPT, characterized by a spectrophotometer. An *in vitro* evaluation showed that these MNPs exhibited toxic behavior toward a fibroblast cell line and breast cancer cells. Therefore, chemotherapy can be enhanced by combining it with PDT [62]. In another study, the microemulsion-based technique was used to create a combination of MNPs and upconversion NPs. The synthesized material was then utilized for two purposes: effective magnetic targeting and the simultaneous production of luminescence by the NPs, thus facilitating PDT. The researchers reported that during *in vivo* NIR imaging, the NPs had a tendency to travel toward and aggregate at the tumor site when the magnet was placed closer to the tumor. Such aggregation was observed to occur six times more in the magnet-treated group. This showed that the MNPs had a significant role in enhancing the PDT [63]. In another study, different photosensitizers based on Cr and Mn MNPs were created, which were combined with curcumin to facilitate PDT. The drug release from Mn MNPs exhibited a higher percentage rate of release under acidic conditions, whereas the release rate from Cr MNPs was the same across different pH values due to the constant surface charge. The nanomaterial was biocompatible, as evaluated by lethal dose determination and hemolysis assay. The cell viability, moreover, confirmed that the efficiency of Mn was higher compared to that of Cr MNPs in PDT [64]. For the treatment of Ehrlich ascites carcinoma, different strategies were evaluated, both individually and in combination. The strategies evaluated included MNPs, PDT laser, direct current electrotherapy, and the anti-cancer drug methotrexate. After investigating all necessary parameters in *in vivo* studies with the aforementioned treatments, they observed that MNP treatment led to the irradiation of tumor cells due to the production of ROS. However, MNPs in combination with the anticancer drug, when exposed to electrotherapy and light, showed the highest antitumor efficiency. This was due to the potent properties of MNPs, which can convert electrotherapy and PDT into magnetic heating that is effective in cancer therapy. Hence, combining all the treatments together yields an efficient therapeutic platform for cancer [65]. Another approach based on MNPs was applied to enhance PDT. A novel nanoplatform was created by the coprecipitation method, which converted the upregulated ROS into free radicals of •OH and O_2 via the Fenton reaction. As a result, the overexpressed oxygen triggered PDT. The researchers reported that light sensitizers were grafted on the surface of the MNPs, which helped in the conversion of the ionic states, leading to the overexpression of oxygen. The oxygen produced in this way served as a raw material for the PDT. In this study, Hou *et al* reported that the mechanism of mitochondrial targeting overcame the inefficiency of ROS production and resulted in tumor cell apoptosis, effectively increasing the PDT effect. Hence, the Fenton reaction could be a novel approach for enhancing PDT [66]. Another example, involving Cerenkov radiation-induced PDT with magnetic target delivery, was reported by Ni *et al.* They fabricated MNPs with radiolabeled Zr and altered them with porphyrin molecules as a surface modifier. The combination of luminescence, energy transfer by Cerenkov radiation, and fluorescence was shown to monitor the therapeutic process. Under the influence of a magnetic field, the MNPs helped this platform to efficiently aggregate in the tumor. Thus, this approach overcame the commercial drawbacks of light- and depth-dependent PDT [67]. The covalent bond between ZnPc complexes and MNPs, which kept the therapeutic materials together during therapy and maximized their efficacy, was highlighted in this study. By targeting folate receptors that frequently occur on tumor cells, this novel strategy sought to enhance PDT efficacy and enable specific targeting. This study suggested that combining MNPs with light sensitizers can result in more potent treatments for cancer, demonstrating this using both magnetic properties for targeted distribution and photodynamic capabilities for generating cytotoxic effects on tumor cells [68]. In another study, MNPs with a customized structure were used to deliver a drug to the tumor site for the treatment of breast cancer. The characteristics of MNPs enabled them to produce oxygen by catalyzing the breakdown of H_2O_2, which improved the distribution of MNPs within tumor cells, thus increasing the overall efficacy of PDT. According to this study, the efficacy of tumor suppression is significantly increased when a magnetic field is applied, indicating an opportunity for the localized treatment of tumors. To further address common issues such as hypoxia and restricted penetration of light sensitizers into tumors, MNPs work together to improve permeation through the thick cellular matrices of solid tumors. In *in vitro* studies, treatment with MNPs led to improved rates of apoptosis and necrosis in 4T1 tumor cells. Through better targeting and increased production of ROS, the integration of MNPs with drug delivery offers a viable approach to improving the therapeutic effectiveness of cancer therapies [69]. Similarly, the sol–gel method was used to synthesize MNPs that were designed for PDT combined with imaging. The magnetic characteristics facilitated the use of MRI for tumor detection. This study also demonstrated how the nanoparticles were successfully modified to increase their zeta value and dispersion stability, suggesting a robust formulation in aqueous solutions. By integrating imaging and therapeutic properties, MNPs solve the problems associated with conventional PDT, such as restricted light penetration, opening an opportunity for novel cancer therapy approaches that make use of magnetically guided deep PDT [70]. In another study, Wang *et al* reported that the physical and biological principles of MNPs improved therapeutic efficacy while lowering systemic adverse effects, marking a major leap in the field of multi-disciplinary cancer treatment [71].

3.6 Magnetic-hyperthermia-based therapy

Magnetic-hyperthermia-based therapy (MHT) has been used as a therapeutic technique for the treatment of solid tumors for decades and is the subject of current clinical studies of the treatment of malignant prostate and brain tumors [72]. The use of MNPs as a therapeutic agent has been shown to improve the efficacy of tumor radiation and thermotherapy [73]. MNPs generate heat through noninvasive methods in response to an imposed magnetic field, allowing them to be used to treat tumor cells [74]. During this process, live cells do not absorb the magnetic field; hence, MNPs can travel inside the body [46]. The ability to inject MNPs directly into a tumor and their production of heat when exposed to a magnetic field results in heat-based shock, ultimately causing cells to undergo apoptosis or necrosis [75]. According to this study, MNPs have high magnetic saturation and persistence in aqueous solutions when treated with biocompatible polymers, which qualifies them for therapeutic uses. Systemic and local routes were investigated; local injections were shown to effectively ablate tumors when paired with a concentrated magnetic field to promote their accumulation at the tumor site. Local administration of MNPs and the resulting MHT result in systemic therapeutic reactions that prevent the spread of tumors. This pairing builds a strong immunological memory, which is essential for avoiding the recurrence of the tumor, in addition to improving the immediate efficacy of tumor treatment. These results highlighted the possibility of employing MNPs as a very successful MHT agent and the encouraging results of combining MHT with immunotherapy to provide systemic therapeutic benefits that endure long after localized treatment [76]. The authors of another study explained that the concept of MHT is that malignant cells can be localized for therapy without causing damage to nearby healthy tissue. The reason for this is that they are more sensitive to temperature rises (usually to temperatures between 42 °C and 45 °C) than normal cells. The researchers used the term ‘intrinsic loss power’, which was the crucial factor that characterized the heating. In their study, the synthesized MNPs exhibited better heating performance when compared to traditional MNPs, resulting in greater performance in MHT. The low toxicity detected in healthy L929 cells indicated how biocompatible these MNPs were, which makes them appropriate for therapeutic uses. The hyaluronic acid coating used in the MNPs improved targeting specificity to tumor cells that overexpress CD44, which is very important for the treatment of breast cancer [77]. In another study, receptor-mediated endocytosis was shown to be responsible for the notable increase in drug accumulation in C6 glioma cells relative to healthy cells when MNPs were employed as carriers for the chemotherapeutic anticancer drug temozolomide (TMZ). Local hyperthermia was generated due to the alteration in the magnetic field, resulting in tumor cell apoptosis due to the increase in temperature, while healthy cells were unaffected. The researchers highlighted that the release of drugs from MNPs is significantly enhanced in the presence of a magnetic field, producing the maximum therapeutic effect. A synergistic effect was created by combining drug-carrying MNPs with a magnetic field, which led to higher toxicity in tumor cells. Hence, they reported a system that allowed controlled release and targeted administration of MNPs, increasing their effectiveness in cancer therapy [78]. Pan *et al* reported the use of zinc-based MNPs for the treatment of liver cancer with MHT. These MNPs were developed to overcome the commercial drawbacks of early elimination by the body's defense system; thus, these MNPs reduced liver immunity, allowing it to retain substances that were intravenously administered. Because of the Zn doping, the MNPs experienced an improved magnetic effect without sacrificing their superparamagnetic characteristics, helping them to be administered intravenously (figure 3.5). By altering these MNPs with a VEGF antibody, which binds to the overexpressed VEGF on these tumor cells, they targeted the HepG2 liver cancer cell line, increasing therapeutic efficacy and minimizing damage to healthy tissues. Even at a mild level, MHT inhibited the proliferation of cancer cells and resulted in apoptosis. In animal models, this approach prolonged survival by suppressing tumor development and improving the immune system's ability to identify and eliminate cancer cells [79]. The findings of another study emphasized how the apoptotic pathways triggered after MHT are strongly influenced by the intracellular amount of MNPs. The intrinsic apoptotic pathway, which is defined by low caspase-8 activity and a high Bax/Bcl-2 mRNA ratio, is mostly activated at lower doses, suggesting a more regulated kind of cellular death. On the other hand, enhanced caspase-8 activity at higher doses indicated an increased level of apoptosis and highlighted the extrinsic route. The dual nature of the apoptotic pathways emphasizes how crucial it is to adjust MNP doses in order to maximize therapeutic effectiveness. The study also highlighted the importance of the intracellular circulation of MNPs, which can vary and impact therapy, and the timing of MNP administration and AMF application. Additionally, the study suggested that the heat generated by MNPs may cause lysosomal membrane permeabilization, which in turn may contribute to cell death [80]. Another report suggested that smaller MNPs produced less heat during Néel relaxation, a feature of superparamagnetic activity, due to lower-energy interactions. The more efficient but size-dependent method of producing heat by larger MNPs is via hysteretic loss. The shift between these two processes is crucial because it establishes the ideal MNP size to provide the highest heating efficiency while preserving treatment safety. Furthermore, the Curie temperature of MNPs is essential for controlling their heat output, since it keeps the temperature below therapeutic thresholds, which normally fall between 42 °C and 45 °C. Investigators are working to improve these characteristics so that MNPs may accurately target tumor tissues and be precisely managed in a non-intrusive way, increasing their heating capacity [81]. MNPs were functionalized in this study, which enhanced their magnetic sensitivity and dispersibility in water. The ability of MNPs to heat up is essential because it dictates how well they may cause cancer cells to overheat. This study showed that the particle size, induced magnetic field, and surface coating collectively influence MNPs' heating efficiency. These nanoparticles demonstrated strong destructive efficacy against the HepG2 liver cancer cell line and high

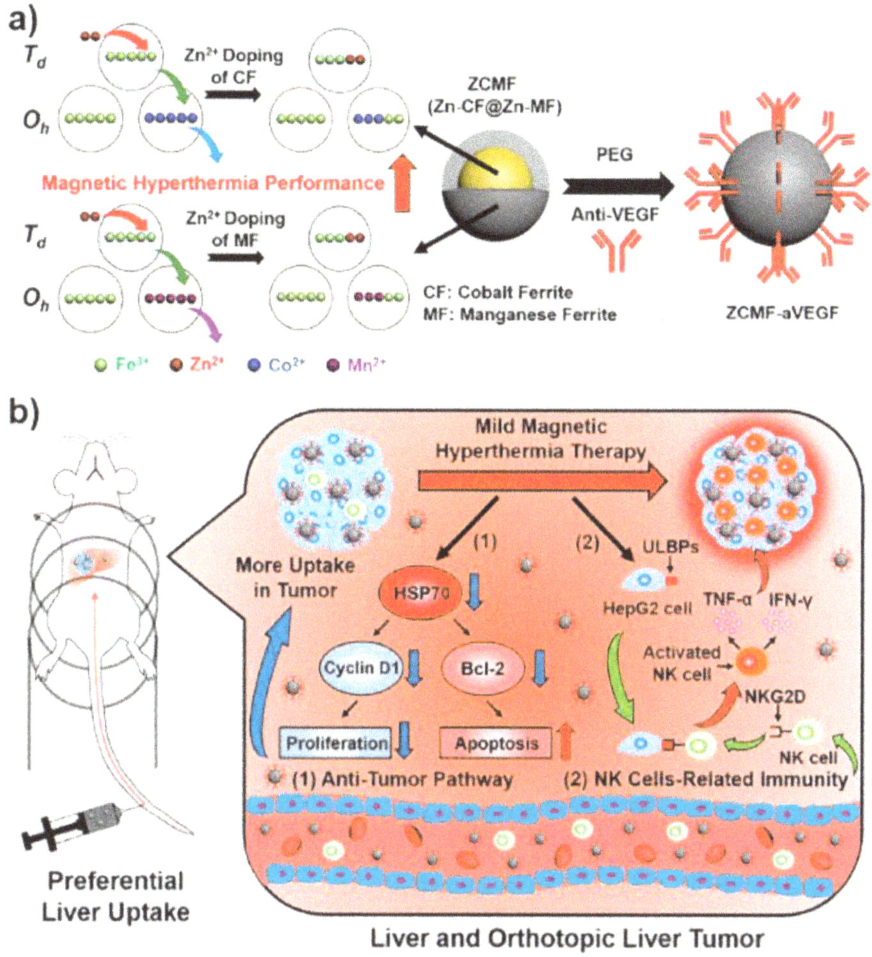

Figure 3.5. Schematics of magnetism enhancements, mild magnetic hyperthermia, and antitumor immunity induction for liver cancer therapy. (a) Illustrations of the synthesis of superparamagnetic nanoparticles, showing Zn^{2+}-doping and the core–shell structure of Zn^{2+}-doped Zn-$CoFe_2O_4$@Zn-$MnFe_2O_4$ (ZCMF) used to enhance magnetism, along with further anti-VEGF modification used to obtain ZCMF-aVEGF. (b) Illustrative presentations of cancer cell proliferation inhibition and natural killer cell activation-related antitumor immunity used for treating orthotopic liver tumors by mild MHT. Adapted with permission from [79]. Copyright (2021) American Chemical Society.

cytocompatibility, confirming their feasibility as potent nanomedicines for tumor thermotherapies [82]. Another report described the synthesis of MNPs with capping agents through various methods, such as coprecipitation, which could be modified using malic and citric acids to improve their effectiveness. In the process of successfully targeting tumor cells, the capping materials not only increased the magnetic strength of the MNPs but also decreased their size. A magnetic field that produced energy when the MNPs were stimulated could be used to control these MNPs due to their special superparamagnetic activity. The cancer cells were effectively damaged by this heat, which caused them to undergo apoptosis. According to studies, the size of tumors significantly decreases when capped MNPs are injected into them and subjected to a magnetic field. This study reported that the capped MNPs, due to their uniform structure, performed better in interactions with tumor cells than uncapped MNPs [83]. According to a further study, a nanocomposite composed of graphene oxide and iron oxide was developed to solve a number of issues with MNPs, including low specific absorption rate and poor colloidal stability. Their stability and biocompatibility were improved by the electrochemical manufacturing technique used, which qualified them for *in vivo* applications. These MNPs possessed a high specific absorption rate, which is important because it determines their conversion of electromagnetic energy into the heat required for MHT. This article presents encouraging *in vitro* findings, demonstrating that at particular temperatures and durations, the nanocomposite caused a notable 80.5% reduction in mortality due to tumors. The results indicate that due to their enhancement of heating efficiency and colloidal integrity, MNPs may become essential to the development of tailored therapies for cancer in the future, providing a less intrusive treatment alternative with potentially fewer adverse effects than conventional techniques [84]. Another study emphasized the use of circular MNPs, 11 nm in size, which were ideal for *in vivo* use because of their superparamagnetic characteristics that inhibited clumping and enabled efficient heating. To improve their absorption by macrophages and cancer cells, which have a substantial need for energy, these MNPs were modified with glucose. Two different 3D tissue culture models were used in the study: (a) one that showed MNPs only inside cells, and (b) another that showed MNPs both within and outside cells. The findings demonstrated the dual function of MNPs in regulating cellular reactions during MHT, with necrosis occurring in model (a) and apoptosis occurring in model (b). The movement of MNPs was shown to have a substantial impact on the processes of cellular destruction. These results imply that MNPs enhance the efficacy of MHT in the treatment of malignancy by acting as a source of extracellular matrix disruption and intrinsic hotspots for targeted heating [85].

3.7 MNPs in cancer theranostics (diagnosis and therapy)

The term ‘magnetotheranostics’ was coined to reflect the capabilities of this approach in both diagnosis and treatment [86]. The treatment, when combined with imaging, amounts to precise therapy, and hence, the effectiveness of a specific treatment can be increased by employing sophisticated imaging techniques to track and evaluate its action against disease [87]. MNPs are perfect theranostic platforms, since they respond to magnetic fields when used in a variety of methods and have integrated capabilities such as magnetism-responsive features [88]. Generally, MNPs are used in positron emission tomography (PET), MRI, PA imaging, ultrasound (US) imaging, computed tomography (CT), optical fluorescence imaging, and single-photon emission computed tomography (SPECT) [89]. By acting as a contrasting agent, MNPs improve MRI contrast and resolution by altering the relaxation times of nearby water protons, and their versatility makes them highly valuable in diagnostic imaging and research applications. Their multimodal potential enables applications that benefit from the strengths of both CT and MRI [90]. Similarly, MNPs support PET imaging by serving as carriers for radioisotopes, enabling multimodal imaging, targeted delivery, and improved localization [91]. MNPs enhance PA imaging by improving optical absorption and signal generation and US imaging through magnet-based acoustic effects and targeted delivery. Thus, their multimodal and theranostic potential makes them highly valuable in advanced imaging and therapeutic applications [92]. For example, Liang *et al* reported the treatment of tumors through PTT under MRI and PA observation. The complex with iron used for the treatment had the potential to absorb under weak acidic pH conditions and exhibited strong magnetic resonance, which was absorbed in the NIR region. This aided in identifying the tumor site, which attracted more laser sources to target the cancer cells. Utilizing the signals of PA and MRI from this complex, the treatment probe was tracked to obtain the doses and the locations of the tumor cells, and the therapy was monitored [93]. In a further study, the fabrication of a nanocluster with a magnetic nature was reported to function as a contrast agent in diagnostic applications. The cavity of this structure that reacted to NIR-II light was hollow, allowing space for the loading of the anticancer drug DOX and further acted as a contrast agent to monitor tumor targeting. The researchers explained the pH-dependent drug release mechanism and, using the Fenton reaction to produce free radicals, subsequently applied chemotherapy. In addition, NIR-II light was transformed to heat by the absorption of the complex, enhancing the release of the drug. Hence, these magnetic clusters provided the combined effect of PTT and chemotherapy with an image-guided platform for cancer therapy [94]. Similarly, Jiang *et al* synthesized MNPs from Mn, which enhanced PTT with a magnetic capability that was used for imaging in a 4T1 breast cancer animal model. They reported that dual-mode imaging, made possible by the Mn-doped MNPs, was capable of determining the presence of a tumor. In *in vitro* and *in vivo* investigations, these MNPs modified by Mn and functionalized by peptide targeting improved tumor signals and reduced the development of cancer cells via PTT provided by magnetic resonance [95]. In another study, Mn and indocyanine green were used to synthesize MNPs, creating a temperature-dependent polymer matrix system (figure 3.6). This system was nontoxic and had the potential to release MNPs under specific laser irradiation, producing a light-induced magnetic MNP system. The researchers reported that continuous heat was produced under a laser light source at 880 nm, which altered the structure of the polymer to emit the Mn MNPs for imaging. The results suggested that the tumor cells had undergone apoptosis due to the production of ROS and generated heat, which caused heat-based swelling in the lysosomes [96]. A multilayered structure was designed for colon cancer treatment using photothermal technology. This structure consisted of SiO_2 shells protecting MNPs for magnetic properties, conjugated with gold NPs, and surface-coated with the anticancer drug cisplatin. This combination of MNPs exhibited strong magnetic resonance during treatment. In addition, they reported that the use of lasers significantly enhanced the irradiation of cancer cells by 50%. The combination of the drug with the gold NPs in the presence of lasers effectively improved the

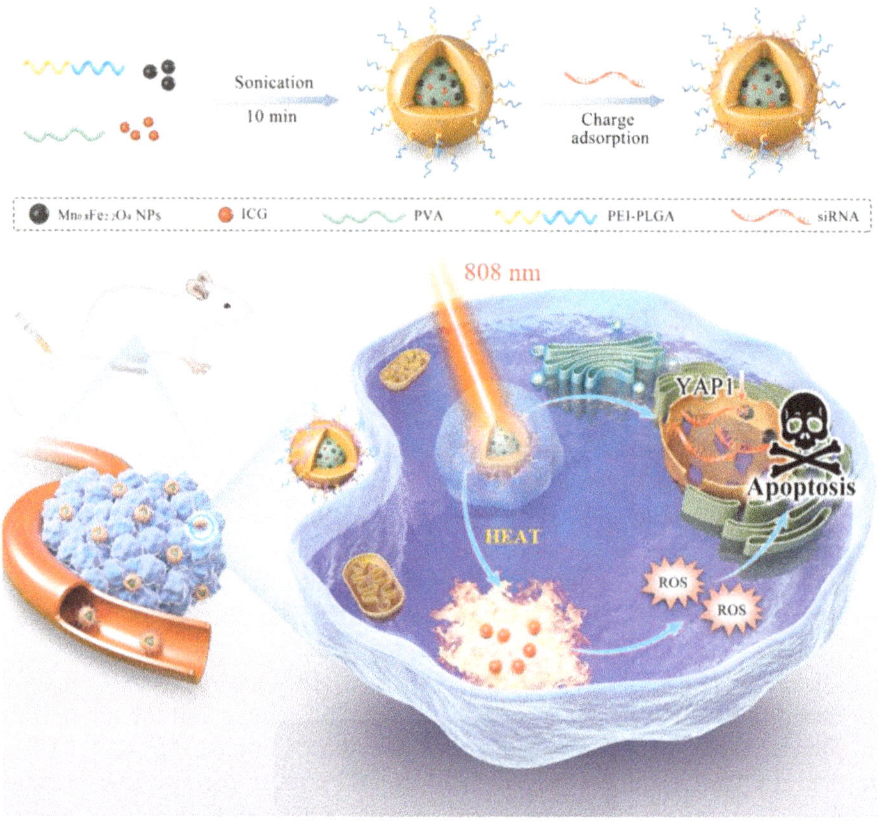

Figure 3.6. Schematic illustration of heat-induced manganese-doped magnetic nanocarriers combined with YAP1 small interfering RNA (siRNA) for MRI/NIR-guided mild PTT therapy of hepatocellular carcinoma and YAP1 regulation. Adapted from [96], Copyright (2021), with permission from Elsevier.

treatment of colon cancer investigated *in vitro* using the SW620 and SW480 cell lines and thus acted as a contrast agent to provide image-guided theranostics [97]. In another study, MNPs designed for magnetic hyperthermia and PT were used to treat cancer in a mouse model. Due to their higher absorption, the NPs used in the NIR region were acceptable for PA imaging. The researchers demonstrated that, at the same molar concentration of Fe, the intensity of magnetic particle imaging using MNPs modified with polyethylene glycol (PEG) increased at a particle size of 10 nm. This signified that MNPs coated with carbon can serve as a sensitive tool for magnetothermal PTT [98]. Chen *et al* reported PDT for breast cancer along with ferroptosis, which was supported by MRI. MNPs made from ferric oxide and chlorin were synthesized and then surface-coated with a poly(lactic-co-glycolic acid) (PLGA) polymer for the therapy. The MNPs reacted and dissociated into ions, producing free radicals and resulting in ferroptosis in the tumor cells. PDT was used to aid in the enhancement of ROS production, followed by the dissociation of chlorin ions under the Fenton reaction. This ROS production enhanced by PDT synergistically encouraged ferroptosis in 4T1 cells. This system suggests that effective suppression of cancer, combined with with an efficient MRI capability, is possible in an animal model with a biocompatible nature [99]. Similarly, a structure with MNPs was created that can target tumor cells in combination with the anticancer drug DOX and FA. These MNPs were able enhance MRI by altering the contrast range and also break down to improve cancer treatment via programmed cell death ferroptosis in the tumor cells. *In vitro* and *in vivo* investigations suggested that this system can provide three different types of therapy all at once, namely ferroptosis, chemotherapy, and PTT in eradicating tumor cells. They further reported that transcription activity and chromatin modification were downregulated, whereas electron transport and respiration inside cells were overexpressed, which ultimately created apoptosis in cells [100]. To enhance NIR imaging and increase cellular uptake while retaining biocompatibility, Li *et al* used a tumor cell coating on the surface of MNPs loaded with a light sensitizer for PDT. The researchers compared coated and uncoated groups and reported the efficiency and potential of the tumor-cell-membrane-coated group compared to the other group. This technique enhanced light-based cytotoxicity to cancer cells under irradiation at 670 nm and increased MRI performance. *In vivo* studies using the SMMC-7721 mouse model suggested that effective PDT was delivered due to the coating process [101]. In another study, Deng *et al.* showed that individual oxygen molecules produced during PDT may be visually detected both *in vitro* and *in vivo* using a synthesized MRI probe. The researchers created an MRI probe from PEG-2000-based micelles using MNPs encapsulated in the light sensitizer Ce6. They reported the use of a specific linker that had the potential to detect a single molecule of evolved oxygen. This linker was cleaved when the light was produced, resulting in a decrease in the PEG concentration present on the surface. Laser irradiation resulted in the accumulation of MNPs and increased hydrophobicity, thus producing oxygen. This evolved oxygen further promoted the MRI signals in the detection of *in vivo* investigations [102]. Similarly, MNPs were created using protoporphyrin IX to dissolve nanoclusters of MNPs without any extra material in such a way that they acted as both a light sensitizer in PDT and a contrast agent in MRI. The protoporphyrin IX enhanced the properties of MNPs in terms of stability, potency, and drug loading, and can be produced on a large scale. *In vivo* investigations suggested that the coating of this material, when treated at 1/8 of the dose, showed a reduction in tumor development in a syngeneic mouse breast cancer model compared to other groups. Hence, the researchers reported that just iron oxide MNPs and protoporphyrin IX, without any further additional material, were stable, low-cost, and effective in image-based therapy of breast cancer [103].

3.8 Combination of therapies using MNPs

In recent years, research has shown the improvement in cancer treatment when a combination of therapies is used; in general terms, these include chemotherapy, radiotherapy, and immunotherapy. The reason for combining more than one therapy is the additive and synergistic effect gained by coupling them [104].

Combining therapies in cancer treatment is a common strategy to enhance efficacy, reduce resistance, and minimize toxicity. Cancer often involves multiple pathways that drive tumor growth and survival. Combining therapies, such as chemotherapy, targeted therapy, and immunotherapy, allows for the simultaneous disruption of multiple mechanisms, making it harder for cancer cells to survive [105]. Tumor cells can develop resistance to single agents over time. Using a combination of drugs with different mechanisms of action reduces the likelihood of resistance by targeting cancer in multiple ways. Some therapies work better together than individually [106]. For example, chemotherapy can increase the effectiveness of immunotherapy by exposing tumor antigens, enhancing the immune system's ability to recognize and attack cancer cells. Tumors are often heterogeneous, containing a mix of cells with different characteristics [107]. Combining therapies results in a broader attack on diverse cell populations within a tumor. Lower doses of each therapy can be used in combination, potentially reducing the toxicity associated with high doses of a single treatment while maintaining or enhancing efficacy [108]. For example, Mn-based MNPs have emerged as a tool in combined cancer therapy, particularly in conjunction with immunotherapy and PTT. In breast cancer models, MNPs showed remarkable effectiveness in halting tumor development and avoiding lung metastases, demonstrating their potential to improve treatment results. Tumor antigen release during PTT facilitates the activation of both general and specific immune responses while downregulating immunosuppressive factors, which is the reason for the efficacy of MNPs. Additionally, these MNPs have demonstrated minimal cytotoxicity while preserving high cell viability, highlighting their safety for use in medicinal settings. Their use in combination successfully counteracts the suppressive microenvironment of the tumor by promoting dendritic cell development and increasing the production of M1-associated cytokines while decreasing M2-associated cytokines. In addition to their therapeutic use, MNPs are useful as contrast agents in MRI, which improves their clinical value and helps diagnose tumors [109]. Another study introduced a new delivery method with MNPs at its core. These NPs efficiently carried the immunostimulator R837 hydrochloride and indocyanine green (ICG) for PTT via a polyethylene glycol polyphenol (DPA-PEG) coating (figure 3.7). By enabling the regulated release of therapeutic drugs, this design increased cancer targeting in the presence of an external magnetic field, which in turn enhanced MNP accumulation at the tumor location. The MNPs created focused hyperthermia in response to NIR irradiation, which caused the destruction of tumors and the release of antigens linked to the malignancy that triggered a response from the immune system. In addition to preventing tumor development, PTT and immunotherapy also address metastasis and recurrence, demonstrating a collaborative effect that increases treatment effectiveness with negligible adverse effects. According to this study, the designed MNPs performed better in animal models at preventing the growth of cancerous cells and enhancing the rate of survival, suggesting that they may find use in clinical cancer treatment [110]. Xiong *et al* reported MNPs, particularly those intended for the combinational therapy of ovarian cancer. By combining red blood cell membranes with ovarian carcinoma cell membranes produced from mice, these MNPs' hybrid biomimetic coating increased their resistance to immune elimination and lengthened their transport period

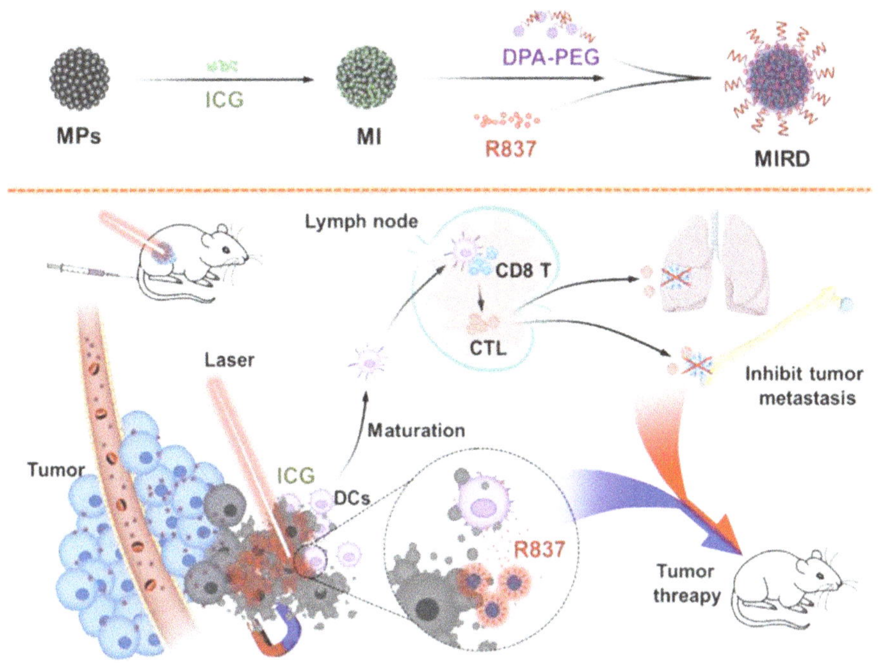

Figure 3.7. Schematic illustration of MIRDs for photothermal/immunotherapy against cancer. Adapted from [110], Copyright (2020), with permission from Elsevier.

in the bloodstream. This study showed that these MNPs effectively suppressed tumor development by retaining the proteins from both types of cells and exhibiting specialized targeting abilities toward the ID8 ovarian cancer cell line. The MNPs facilitated PTT, which raised the temperature at the location of the tumor to levels high enough to destroy cancerous cells when combined with NIR irradiation. The response of the immune system to the carcinoma was further strengthened by this heat impact, which also made it easier for whole-cell antigens of the tumor to be released. The presence of increased numbers of CD8+ cytotoxic T cells and decreased numbers of regulatory T cells in the tumor microenvironment demonstrated that the combination of PTT and immunotherapy enhanced anticancer effects. In order to minimize off-target effects, the study demonstrated that MNPs can successfully target related cancer cells while preserving non-target cells, hence activating targeted immunity [111]. Another article reported that utilizing these MNPs as drug delivery systems can improve tailored delivery to cancer locations, particularly when paired with external magnetic modulation that permits specific retention at the tumor site. The ejection of iron ions from MNPs is facilitated by the acidic environment of the tumor surroundings. The Fenton reaction can produce ROS, aiding in chemodynamic treatment. However, issues such as the propensity of MNPs to undergo oxidation and agglomerate might make them less secure and efficient for intravenous administration. Strategies such as hiding MNPs inside cell membranes and operational alterations have been investigated to solve these problems; however, these techniques may be intricate and involve hazardous chemicals. This work demonstrated that gold nanoparticles may successfully functionalize magnetosome membranes *in situ*, forming a core–satellite system that improves detection and effectiveness in therapy. These modified MNPs exhibited notable increases in tumor cell cytotoxicity when used in conjunction with chemodynamic, photothermal, and starvation treatments. This was particularly evident in acidic environments and when laser radiation was used, which resulted in almost total suppression of tumor cell development. Additionally, *in vivo* research showed that MNPs can successfully stop tumor development in a variety of xenograft models, highlighting their potential use in novel cancer treatment strategies [112]. For example, MNPs such as manganese ferrite have been developed to serve as both photosensitizers and sonosensitizers in the treatment of cancer, as well as contrast agents for MRI. When MNPs are used in treatment, ultrasonic waves and NIR light can be used, activating the MNPs to produce heat or ROS that efficiently kill the cancerous cells. Studies have demonstrated that PTT and sonodynamic therapy (SDT) delivered by MNPs operate in conjunction to overcome the drawbacks of each separate treatment; thus, this combination can result in notable tumor shrinkage. Furthermore, the capacity of MNPs to deeply permeate into the tissues improves the therapeutic impact on malignancies that would otherwise be challenging to treat because of restrictions in light penetration. A number of studies have shown that MNPs are biocompatible, which enhances their potential for clinical use by enabling efficient therapy with few adverse effects [113]. In another study, MNPs were used to produce a dual-purpose nanocomposite MHT effect using the photosensitizing qualities of curcumin. The goal of this strategy was to overcome the drawbacks of utilizing either PDT or PTT alone, which frequently leads to less-than-ideal treatment results for reasons such as a lack of photosensitizer solubility or the inadequate targeting of cancer cells. By adding MNPs, therapeutic drugs may be delivered simultaneously, and an external magnetic field can be applied to guide the MNPs to the lesion location, improving the accuracy and efficacy of therapy. The combination of NC, PTT, and PDT achieved an impressive 27% drop in tumor density compared to its original volume, demonstrating the promise of this method in curing breast cancer. This study also showed that pairing MNPs with PDT and PTT resulted in substantial decreases in carcinoma volume. Additionally, the application of MNPs promoted the production of ROS and hyperthermia at the tumor site, both of which are essential for triggering the death of cancer cells. According to the results, MNPs are a useful tool in the battle against illnesses, since they not only increase the distribution and production of photosensitizers but also boost the overall curative efficiency of combination therapy strategies [114].

References

[1] Li X, Li W, Wang M and Liao Z 2021 Magnetic nanoparticles for cancer theranostics: advances and prospects *J. Control. Release* **335** 437–48

[2] Ferreira M, Sousa J, Pais A and Vitorino C 2020 The role of magnetic nanoparticles in cancer nanotheranostics *Materials* **13** 266

[3] Mukherjee S, Liang L and Veiseh O 2020 Recent advancements of magnetic nanomaterials in cancer therapy *Pharmaceutics* **12** 147

[4] Sharma K and Chauhan C 2023 Role of magnetic nanoparticle (MNPs) in cancer treatment: a review *Mater. Today Proc.* **81** 919–25

[5] Anjum T, Hussain N, Iqbal H M, Jedrzak A, Jesionowski T and Bilal M 2023 Magnetic nanomaterials as drug delivery vehicles and therapeutic constructs to treat cancer *J. Drug Deliv. Sci. Technol.* **80** 104103

[6] Senapati S, Mahanta A K, Kumar S and Maiti P 2018 Controlled drug delivery vehicles for cancer treatment and their performance *Signal Transduct. Target. Ther.* **3** 7

[7] Aslam H, Shukrullah S, Naz M Y, Fatima H, Hussain H, Ullah S and Assiri M A 2022 Current and future perspectives of multifunctional magnetic nanoparticles based controlled drug delivery systems *J. Drug Deliv. Sci. Technol.* **67** 102946

[8] Albinali K E, Zagho M M, Deng Y and Elzatahry A A 2019 A perspective on magnetic core–shell carriers for responsive and targeted drug delivery systems *Int. J. Nanomed.* **14** 1707–23

[9] Kim D I, Lee H, Kwon S H, Sung Y J, Song W K and Park S 2020 Bilayer hydrogel sheet-type intraocular microrobot for drug delivery and magnetic nanoparticles retrieval *Adv. Healthc. Mater.* **9** 2000118

[10] Lee H, Kim D-i, Kwon S-h and Park S 2021 Magnetically actuated drug delivery helical microrobot with magnetic nanoparticle retrieval ability *ACS Appl. Mater. Interfaces* **13** 19633–47

[11] Han H, Hou Y, Chen X, Zhang P, Kang M, Jin Q, Ji J and Gao M 2020 Metformin-induced stromal depletion to enhance the penetration of gemcitabine-loaded magnetic nanoparticles for pancreatic cancer targeted therapy *J. Am. Chem. Soc.* **142** 4944–54

[12] Taherian A, Esfandiari N and Rouhani S 2021 Breast cancer drug delivery by novel drug-loaded chitosan-coated magnetic nanoparticles *Cancer Nanotechnol.* **12** 1–20

[13] Dhavale R P, Dhavale R, Sahoo S, Kollu P, Jadhav S, Patil P, Dongale T, Chougale A and Patil P 2021 Chitosan coated magnetic nanoparticles as carriers of anticancer drug Telmisartan: pH-responsive controlled drug release and cytotoxicity studies *J. Phys. Chem. Solids* **148** 109749

[14] Fathi M, Barar J, Erfan-Niya H and Omidi Y 2020 Methotrexate-conjugated chitosan-grafted pH-and thermo-responsive magnetic nanoparticles for targeted therapy of ovarian cancer *Int. J. Biol. Macromol.* **154** 1175–84

[15] Ebadi M, Buskaran K, Bullo S, Hussein M Z, Fakurazi S and Pastorin G 2021 Drug delivery system based on magnetic iron oxide nanoparticles coated with (polyvinyl alcohol–zinc/aluminium-layered double hydroxide-sorafenib) *Alex. Eng. J.* **60** 733–47

[16] Avedian N, Zaaeri F, Daryasari M P, Javar H A and Khoobi M 2018 pH-sensitive biocompatible mesoporous magnetic nanoparticles labeled with folic acid as an efficient carrier for controlled anticancer drug delivery *J. Drug Deliv. Sci. Technol.* **44** 323–32

[17] Yenurkar D, Nayak M and Mukherjee S 2023 Recent advances of nanocrystals in cancer theranostics *Nanoscale Adv.* **5** 4018–40

[18] Rosenblum D, Joshi N, Tao W, Karp J M and Peer D 2018 Progress and challenges towards targeted delivery of cancer therapeutics *Nat. Commun.* **9** 1410

[19] Saepudin E, Fadhilah H R and Khalil M 2020 The influence of carboxylate moieties for efficient loading and pH-controlled release of doxorubicin in Fe_3O_4 magnetic nanoparticles *Colloids Surf.,* A **602** 125137

[20] Solak K, Mavi A and Yılmaz B 2021 Disulfiram-loaded functionalized magnetic nanoparticles combined with copper and sodium nitroprusside in breast cancer cells *Mater. Sci. Eng.* C **119** 111452

[21] Ahmadi S, Fazilati M, Nazem H and Mousavi S M 2021 Green synthesis of magnetic nanoparticles using *Satureja hortensis* essential oil toward superior antibacterial/fungal and anticancer performance *BioMed Res. Int.* **2021** 8822645

[22] Yıldırım M, Acet Ö, Acet B Ö, Karakoç V and Odabaşı M 2024 Innovative approach against cancer: thymoquinone-loaded PHEMA-based magnetic nanoparticles and their effects on MCF-7 breast cancer *Biochem. Biophys. Res. Commun.* **734** 150464

[23] Alavi O, Babavalian H, Shakeri F, Hashemzadeh M S and Nemati M M 2024 Synthesis and evaluation of the anticancer effects of iron oxide-chitosan magnetic nanoparticles loaded atorvastatin on the invasion and tumorigenicity of C6 cell line in glioblastoma animal model *J. Polym. Environ.* **32** 6742–59

[24] Jabir M S, Nayef U M, Abdulkadhim W K and Sulaiman G M 2019 Supermagnetic Fe_3O_4-PEG nanoparticles combined with NIR laser and alternating magnetic field as potent anticancer agent against human ovarian cancer cells *Mater. Res. Express* **6** 115412

[25] Cheng H W, Tsao H Y, Chiang C S and Chen S Y 2021 Advances in magnetic nanoparticle-mediated cancer immune-theranostics *Adv. Healthc. Mater.* **10** 2001451

[26] Rahmat J N, Liu J, Chen T, Li Z and Zhang Y 2024 Engineered biological nanoparticles as nanotherapeutics for tumor immunomodulation *Chem. Soc. Rev.* **53** 5862–903

[27] Song Q, Javid A, Zhang G and Li Y 2021 Applications of magnetite nanoparticles in cancer immunotherapies: present hallmarks and future perspectives *Front. Immunol.* **12** 701485

[28] Sau S, Alsaab H O, Bhise K, Alzhrani R, Nabil G and Iyer A K 2018 Multifunctional nanoparticles for cancer immunotherapy: a groundbreaking approach for reprogramming malfunctioned tumor environment *J. Control. Release* **274** 24–34

[29] Day N B, Wixson W C and Shields IV C W 2021 Magnetic systems for cancer immunotherapy *Acta Pharm. Sinica* B **11** 2172–96

[30] Wang S, Wang Z, Li Z, Xu J, Meng X, Zhao Z and Hou Y 2022 A catalytic immune activator based on magnetic nanoparticles to reprogram the immunoecology of breast cancer from 'cold' to 'hot' state *Adv. Healthc. Mater.* **11** 2201240

[31] Lafuente-Gómez N, Wang S, Fontana F, Dhanjani M, García-Soriano D, Correia A, Castellanos M, Diaz C R, Salas G and Santos H A 2022 Synergistic immunomodulatory effect in macrophages mediated by magnetic nanoparticles modified with miRNAs *Nanoscale* **14** 11129–38

[32] Jiang Q, Wang K, Zhang X, Ouyang B, Liu H, Pang Z and Yang W 2020 Platelet membrane-camouflaged magnetic nanoparticles for ferroptosis-enhanced cancer immunotherapy *Small* **16** 2001704

[33] Rao L, Zhao S K, Wen C, Tian R, Lin L, Cai B, Sun Y, Kang F, Yang Z and He L 2020 Activating macrophage-mediated cancer immunotherapy by genetically edited nanoparticles *Adv. Mater.* **32** 2004853

[34] Darya G H, Zare O, Karbalaei-Heidari H R, Zeinali S, Sheardown H and Rastegari B 2024 Enzyme-responsive mannose-grafted magnetic nanoparticles for breast and liver cancer therapy and tumor-associated macrophage immunomodulation *Expert Opin. Drug Deliv.* **21** 663–77

[35] Su Y, Yang F, Wang M and Cheung P C 2023 Cancer immunotherapeutic effect of carboxymethylated β-d-glucan coupled with iron oxide nanoparticles via reprogramming tumor-associated macrophages *Int. J. Biol. Macromol.* **228** 692–705

[36] Jiang H, Fu H, Min T, Hu P and Shi J 2023 Magnetic-manipulated NK cell proliferation and activation enhance immunotherapy of orthotopic liver cancer *J. Am. Chem. Soc.* **145** 13147–60

[37] Wu D, Shou X, Zhang Y, Li Z, Wu G, Wu D, Wu J, Shi S and Wang S 2021 Cell membrane-encapsulated magnetic nanoparticles for enhancing natural killer cell-mediated cancer immunotherapy *Nanomed. Nanotechnol. Biol. Med.* **32** 102333

[38] Gondan A I B, Ruiz-de-Angulo A, Zabaleta A, Blanco N G, Cobaleda-Siles B M, García-Granda M J, Padro D, Llop J, Arnaiz B and Gato M 2018 Effective cancer immunotherapy in mice by polyIC-imiquimod complexes and engineered magnetic nanoparticles *Biomaterials* **170** 95–115

[39] Chiang C-S, Lin Y-J, Lee R, Lai Y-H, Cheng H-W, Hsieh C-H, Shyu W-C and Chen S-Y 2018 Combination of fucoidan-based magnetic nanoparticles and immunomodulators enhances tumour-localized immunotherapy *Nat. Nanotechnol.* **13** 746–54

[40] Traini G, Ruiz-de-Angulo A, Blanco-Canosa J B, Zamacola Bascaran K, Molinaro A, Silipo A, Escors D and Mareque-Rivas J C 2019 Cancer immunotherapy of TLR4 agonist–antigen constructs enhanced with pathogen-mimicking magnetite nanoparticles and checkpoint blockade of PD-L1 *Small* **15** 1803993

[41] Ge R, Liu C, Zhang X, Wang W, Li B, Liu J, Liu Y, Sun H, Zhang D and Hou Y 2018 Photothermal-activatable Fe_3O_4 superparticle nanodrug carriers with PD-L1 immune checkpoint blockade for anti-metastatic cancer immunotherapy *ACS Appl. Mater. Interfaces* **10** 20342–55

[42] Grifantini R, Taranta M, Gherardini L, Naldi I, Parri M, Grandi A, Giannetti A, Tombelli S, Lucarini G and Ricotti L 2018 Magnetically driven drug delivery systems improving targeted immunotherapy for colon-rectal cancer *J. Control. Release* **280** 76–86

[43] Van de Walle A, Figuerola A, Espinosa A, Abou-Hassan A, Estrader M and Wilhelm C 2023 Emergence of magnetic nanoparticles in photothermal and ferroptotic therapies *Mater. Horizons* **10** 4757–75

[44] Xiong Y, Rao Y, Hu J, Luo Z and Chen C 2023 Nanoparticle-based photothermal therapy for breast cancer noninvasive treatment *Adv. Mater.* 2305140

[45] Khizar S, Elkalla E, Zine N, Jaffrezic-Renault N, Errachid A and Elaissari A 2023 Magnetic nanoparticles: multifunctional tool for cancer therapy *Exp. Opin. Drug Deliv.* **20** 189–204

[46] Roy I 2022 Therapeutic applications of magnetic nanoparticles: recent advances *Mater. Adv.* **3** 7425–44

[47] Zhang X, Li Z, Gao J, Wang Z, Gao X, Liu N, Li M, Zhang H and Zheng A 2020 Preparation of nanocrystals for insoluble drugs by top-down nanotechnology with improved solubility and bioavailability *Molecules (Basel, Switzerland)* **25** 1080

[48] Sikora-Dobrowolska B, Borodziuk A, Kulpa-Greszta M, Pazik R, Wojciechowski T, Sobczak K, Rybusinski J, Szczytko J and Klopotowski L 2024 Opto-magnetic nanoparticles with upconverting properties for optical imaging and photothermal therapies *J. Magn. Magn. Mater.* **591** 171714

[49] Zhang L, Li W, Parvin R, Wang X, Fan Q and Ye F 2022 Screening prostate cancer cell-derived exosomal microRNA expression with photothermal-driven digital PCR *Adv. Funct. Mater.* **32** 2207879

[50] Jędrzak A, Grześkowiak B F, Golba K, Coy E, Synoradzki K, Jurga S, Jesionowski T and Mrówczyński R 2020 Magnetite nanoparticles and spheres for chemo-and photothermal therapy of hepatocellular carcinoma *in vitro Int. J. Nanomed.* **15** 7923–36

[51] Sharifi M, Hasan A, Nanakali N M Q, Salihi A, Qadir F A, Muhammad H A, Shekha M S, Aziz F M, Amen K M and Najafi F 2020 Combined chemo-magnetic field-photothermal breast cancer therapy based on porous magnetite nanospheres *Sci. Rep.* **10** 5925

[52] Wang S, Shen H, Mao Q, Tao Q, Yuan G, Zeng L, Chen Z, Zhang Y, Cheng L and Zhang J 2021 Macrophage-mediated porous magnetic nanoparticles for multimodal imaging and postoperative photothermal therapy of gliomas *ACS Appl. Mater. Interfaces* **13** 56825–37

[53] Ji Y and Wang C 2023 Magnetic iron oxide nanoparticle-loaded hydrogels for photothermal therapy of cancer cells *Front. Bioeng. Biotechnol.* **11** 1130523

[54] Lázaro M, Delgado Á V and Iglesias G R 2024 Magneto-photothermal synergy applied to gold-coated magnetic nanoparticles *J. Magn. Magn. Mater.* **591** 171718

[55] Bu L L, Rao L, Yu G T, Chen L, Deng W W, Liu J F, Wu H, Meng Q F, Guo S S and Zhao X Z 2019 Cancer stem cell-platelet hybrid membrane-coated magnetic nanoparticles for enhanced photothermal therapy of head and neck squamous cell carcinoma *Adv. Funct. Mater.* **29** 1807733

[56] Wang Y, Wei G, Zhang X, Huang X, Zhao J, Guo X and Zhou S 2018 Multistage targeting strategy using magnetic composite nanoparticles for synergism of photothermal therapy and chemotherapy *Small* **14** 1702994

[57] Wang L, Chen S, Zhu Y, Zhang M, Tang S, Li J, Pei W, Huang B and Niu C 2018 Triple-modal imaging-guided chemo-photothermal synergistic therapy for breast cancer with magnetically targeted phase-shifted nanoparticles *ACS Appl. Mater. Interfaces* **10** 42102–14

[58] Wang H, Mu Q, Revia R, Wang K, Tian B, Lin G, Lee W, Hong Y-K and Zhang M 2018 Iron oxide-carbon core-shell nanoparticles for dual-modal imaging-guided photothermal therapy *J. Control. Release* **289** 70–8

[59] Ren X, Chen Y, Peng H, Fang X, Zhang X, Chen Q, Wang X, Yang W and Sha X 2018 Blocking autophagic flux enhances iron oxide nanoparticle photothermal therapeutic efficiency in cancer treatment *ACS Appl. Mater. Interfaces* **10** 27701–11

[60] Liu H, Zhang M, Jin H, Tao K, Tang C, Fan Y, Liu S, Liu Y, Hou Y and Zhang H 2022 Fe (III)-doped polyaminopyrrole nanoparticle for imaging-guided photothermal therapy of bladder cancer *ACS Biomater. Sci. Eng.* **8** 502–11

[61] Dinc R 2024 Magnetic nanoparticles with aspects of their use in cancer therapy *Lett. Drug Des. Discov.* **21** 847–57

[62] Vinothini K, Rajendran N K, Rajan M, Ramu A, Marraiki N and Elgorban A M 2020 A magnetic nanoparticle functionalized reduced graphene oxide-based drug carrier system for a chemo-photodynamic cancer therapy *New J. Chem.* **44** 5265–77

[63] Liu Y, Liang Y, Lei P, Zhang Z and Chen Y 2023 Multifunctional superparticles for magnetically targeted NIR-II imaging and photodynamic therapy *Adv. Sci.* **10** 2203669

[64] Aghajanzadeh M, Naderi E, Zamani M, Sharafi A, Naseri M and Danafar H 2020 *In vivo* and *in vitro* biocompatibility study of $MnFe_2O_4$ and $Cr_2Fe_6O_{12}$ as photosensitizer for photodynamic therapy and drug delivery of anti-cancer drugs *Drug Dev. Ind. Pharm.* **46** 846–51

[65] Abo-Neima S E and Elsehly E M 2022 Cancer treatment by laser and electrochemical therapy combined with magnetic nanoparticles as potent therapy against ehrlich ascites carcinoma *BioNanoScience* **12** 851–66

[66] Hou H, Huang X, Wei G, Xu F, Wang Y and Zhou S 2019 Fenton reaction-assisted photodynamic therapy for cancer with multifunctional magnetic nanoparticles *ACS Appl. Mater. Interfaces* **11** 29579–92

[67] Ni D, Ferreira C A, Barnhart T E, Quach V, Yu B, Jiang D, Wei W, Liu H, Engle J W and Hu P 2018 Magnetic targeting of nanotheranostics enhances cerenkov radiation-induced photodynamic therapy *J. Am. Chem. Soc.* **140** 14971–9

[68] Matlou G G, Oluwole D O, Prinsloo E and Nyokong T 2018 Photodynamic therapy activity of zinc phthalocyanine linked to folic acid and magnetic nanoparticles *J. Photochem. Photobiol.,* B **186** 216–24

[69] Zhang P, Wu G, Zhao C, Zhou L, Wang X and Wei S 2020 Magnetic stomatocyte-like nanomotor as photosensitizer carrier for photodynamic therapy based cancer treatment *Colloids Surf.,* B **194** 111204

[70] Jain A, Koyani R, Muñoz C, Sengar P, Contreras O E, Juárez P and Hirata G A 2018 Magnetic-luminescent cerium-doped gadolinium aluminum garnet nanoparticles for simultaneous imaging and photodynamic therapy of cancer cells *J. Colloid Interface Sci.* **526** 220–9

[71] Wang Z, Zhang F, Shao D, Chang Z, Wang L, Hu H, Zheng X, Li X, Chen F and Tu Z 2019 Janus nanobullets combine photodynamic therapy and magnetic hyperthermia to potentiate synergetic anti-metastatic immunotherapy *Adv. Sci.* **6** 1901690

[72] Yu X, Ding S, Yang R, Wu C and Zhang W 2021 Research progress on magnetic nanoparticles for magnetic induction hyperthermia of malignant tumor *Ceram. Int.* **47** 5909–17

[73] Gavilán H, Avugadda S K, Fernández-Cabada T, Soni N, Cassani M, Mai B T, Chantrell R and Pellegrino T 2021 Magnetic nanoparticles and clusters for magnetic hyperthermia: Optimizing their heat performance and developing combinatorial therapies to tackle cancer *Chem. Soc. Rev.* **50** 11614–67

[74] Farzanegan Z and Tahmasbi M 2023 Evaluating the applications and effectiveness of magnetic nanoparticle-based hyperthermia for cancer treatment: a systematic review *Appl. Radiat. Isot.* **198** 110873

[75] Ahmed S, Rajak B L, Gogoi M and Sarma H D 2020 Magnetic nanoparticles mediated cancer hyperthermia *Smart Healthcare for Disease Diagnosis and Prevention* (Amsterdam: Elsevier) 153–73

[76] Chao Y, Chen G, Liang C, Xu J, Dong Z, Han X, Wang C and Liu Z 2019 Iron nanoparticles for low-power local magnetic hyperthermia in combination with immune checkpoint blockade for systemic antitumor therapy *Nano Lett.* **19** 4287–96

[77] Soleymani M, Velashjerdi M, Shaterabadi Z and Barati A 2020 One-pot preparation of hyaluronic acid-coated iron oxide nanoparticles for magnetic hyperthermia therapy and targeting CD44-overexpressing cancer cells *Carbohydr. Polym.* **237** 116130

[78] Minaei S E, Khoei S, Khoee S, Vafashoar F and Mahabadi V P 2019 *In vitro* anti-cancer efficacy of multi-functionalized magnetite nanoparticles combining alternating magnetic hyperthermia in glioblastoma cancer cells *Mater. Sci. Eng.* C **101** 575–87

[79] Pan J, Xu Y, Wu Q, Hu P and Shi J 2021 Mild magnetic hyperthermia-activated innate immunity for liver cancer therapy *J. Am. Chem. Soc.* **143** 8116–28

[80] Beola L, Asín L, Roma-Rodrigues C, Fernández-Afonso Y, Fratila R M, Serantes D, Ruta S, Chantrell R W, Fernandes A R and Baptista P V 2020 The intracellular number of magnetic nanoparticles modulates the apoptotic death pathway after magnetic hyperthermia treatment *ACS Appl. Mater. Interfaces* **12** 43474–87

[81] Shaterabadi Z, Nabiyouni G and Soleymani M 2018 Physics responsible for heating efficiency and self-controlled temperature rise of magnetic nanoparticles in magnetic hyperthermia therapy *Prog. Biophys. Mol. Biol.* **133** 9–19

[82] Kandasamy G, Sudame A, Luthra T, Saini K and Maity D 2018 Functionalized hydrophilic superparamagnetic iron oxide nanoparticles for magnetic fluid hyperthermia application in liver cancer treatment *ACS Omega* **3** 3991–4005

[83] Munir T, Mahmood A, Fakhar-e-Alam M, Imran M, Sohail A, Amin N, Latif S, Rasool H G, Shafiq F and Ali H 2019 Treatment of breast cancer with capped magnetic-NPs induced hyperthermia therapy *J. Mol. Struct.* **1196** 88–95

[84] Kumar R, Chauhan A, Jha S K and Kuanr B K 2018 Localized cancer treatment by radio-frequency hyperthermia using magnetic nanoparticles immobilized on graphene oxide: from novel synthesis to *in vitro* studies *J. Mater. Chem.* B **6** 5385–99

[85] Beola L, Asín L, Fratila R M, Herrero V, Grazú V and Gutiérrez L 2018 Dual role of magnetic nanoparticles as intracellular hotspots and extracellular matrix disruptors triggered by magnetic hyperthermia in 3D cell culture models *Appl. Mater. Interfaces* **10** 44301–13

[86] Liu X, Zhang H, Zhang T, Wang Y, Jiao W, Lu X, Gao X, Xie M, Shan Q and Wen N 2021 Magnetic nanomaterials-mediated cancer diagnosis and therapy *Prog. Biomed. Eng.* **4** 012005

[87] Martinkova P, Brtnicky M, Kynicky J and Pohanka M 2018 Iron oxide nanoparticles: innovative tool in cancer diagnosis and therapy *Adv. Healthc. Mater.* **7** 1700932

[88] Tong S, Zhu H and Bao G 2019 Magnetic iron oxide nanoparticles for disease detection and therapy *Mater. Today* **31** 86–99

[89] Farzin A, Etesami S A, Quint J, Memic A and Tamayol A 2020 Magnetic nanoparticles in cancer therapy and diagnosis *Adv. Healthc. Mater.* **9** 1901058

[90] Aslan N, Ceylan B, Koç M M and Findik F 2020 Metallic nanoparticles as *x*-ray computed tomography (CT) contrast agents: a review *J. Mol. Struct.* **1219** 128599

[91] Liu H, Wang R, Gao H, Chen L, Li X, Yu X, Wu Y, Bai Y, Wei W and Wang M 2024 Nanoprobes for PET/MR imaging *Adv. Therap.* **7** 2300232

[92] Józefczak A, Kaczmarek K and Bielas R 2021 Magnetic mediators for ultrasound theranostics *Theranostics* **11** 10091

[93] Liang G, Han J and Xing D 2021 Precise tumor photothermal therapy guided and monitored by magnetic resonance/photoacoustic imaging using a safe and pH-responsive Fe (III) complex *Adv. Healthc. Mater.* **10** 2001300

[94] Wang X, Li C, Qian J, Lv X, Li H, Zou J, Zhang J, Meng X, Liu H and Qian Y 2021 NIR-II responsive hollow magnetite nanoclusters for targeted magnetic resonance imaging-guided photothermal/chemo-therapy and chemodynamic therapy *Small* **17** 2100794

[95] Jiang G, Fan D, Tian J, Xiang Z and Fang Q 2022 Self-confirming magnetosomes for tumor-targeted T1/T2 dual-mode mri and mri-guided photothermal therapy *Adv. Healthc. Mater.* **11** 2200841

[96] Zhang Q, Zhao W, Cheng J, Deng Z, Zhang P, Zhang A, Xu Z, Pan S, Liao X and Cui D 2021 Heat-induced manganese-doped magnetic nanocarriers combined with Yap-siRNA for MRI/NIR-guided mild photothermal and gene therapy of hepatocellular carcinoma *Chem. Eng. J.* **426** 130746

[97] Maximenko A, Depciuch J, Łopuszyńska N, Stec M, Świątkowska-Warkocka Ż, Bayev V, Zieliński P M, Baran J, Fedotova J and Węglarz W P 2020 Fe_3O_4@ SiO_2@Au nanoparticles for MRI-guided chemo/NIR photothermal therapy of cancer cells *RSC Adv.* **10** 26508–20

[98] Song G, Kenney M, Chen Y-S, Zheng X, Deng Y, Chen Z, Wang S X, Gambhir S S, Dai H and Rao J 2020 Carbon-coated FeCo nanoparticles as sensitive magnetic-particle-imaging tracers with photothermal and magnetothermal properties *Nat. Biomed. Eng.* **4** 325–34

[99] Chen Q, Ma X, Xie L, Chen W, Xu Z, Song E, Zhu X and Song Y 2021 Iron-based nanoparticles for MR imaging-guided ferroptosis in combination with photodynamic therapy to enhance cancer treatment *Nanoscale* **13** 4855–70

[100] Yang B, Zhang Y, Sun L, Wang J, Zhao Z, Huang Z, Mao W, Xue R, Chen R and Luo J 2023 Modulated ultrasmall γ-Fe_2O_3 nanocrystal assemblies for switchable magnetic resonance imaging and photothermal-ferroptotic-chemical synergistic cancer therapy *Adv. Funct. Mater.* **33** 2211251

[101] Li J, Wang X, Zheng D, Lin X, Wei Z, Zhang D, Li Z, Zhang Y, Wu M and Liu X 2018 Cancer cell membrane-coated magnetic nanoparticles for MR/NIR fluorescence dual-modal imaging and photodynamic therapy *Biomater. Sci.* **6** 1834–45

[102] Deng K, Wu B, Wang C X, Wang Q, Yu H, Li J M, Li K H, Zhao H Y and Huang S W 2020 An oxidation-enhanced magnetic resonance imaging probe for visual and specific detection of singlet oxygen generated in photodynamic cancer therapy *in vivo Adv. Healthc. Mater.* **9** 2000533

[103] Yan L, Amirshaghaghi A, Huang D, Miller J, Stein J M, Busch T M, Cheng Z and Tsourkas A 2018 Protoporphyrin IX (PpIX)-coated superparamagnetic iron oxide nanoparticle (SPION) nanoclusters for magnetic resonance imaging and photodynamic therapy *Adv. Funct. Mater.* **28** 1707030

[104] Chowdhury P, Chamoto K and Honjo T 2018 Combination therapy strategies for improving PD-1 blockade efficacy: a new era in cancer immunotherapy *J. Int. Med.* **283** 110–20

[105] Lee A and Djamgoz M B 2018 Triple negative breast cancer: emerging therapeutic modalities and novel combination therapies *Cancer Treat. Rev.* **62** 110–22

[106] Patel S A and Minn A J 2018 Combination cancer therapy with immune checkpoint blockade: mechanisms and strategies *Immunity* **48** 417–33

[107] Gu Z, Zhu S, Yan L, Zhao F and Zhao Y 2019 Graphene-based smart platforms for combined cancer therapy *Adv. Mater.* **31** 1800662

[108] Liang P, Ballou B, Lv X, Si W, Bruchez M P, Huang W and Dong X 2021 Monotherapy and combination therapy using anti-angiogenic nanoagents to fight cancer *Adv. Mater.* **33** 2005155

[109] Zhou B, Wu Q, Wang M, Hoover A, Wang X, Zhou F, Towner R A, Smith N, Saunders D and Song J 2020 Immunologically modified $MnFe_2O_4$ nanoparticles to synergize photothermal therapy and immunotherapy for cancer treatment *Chem. Eng. J.* **396** 125239

[110] Zhang F, Lu G, Wen X, Li F, Ji X, Li Q, Wu M, Cheng Q, Yu Y and Tang J 2020 Magnetic nanoparticles coated with polyphenols for spatio-temporally controlled cancer photothermal/immunotherapy *J. Control. Release* **326** 131–9

[111] Xiong J, Wu M, Chen J, Liu Y, Chen Y, Fan G, Liu Y, Cheng J, Wang Z and Wang S 2021 Cancer-erythrocyte hybrid membrane-camouflaged magnetic nanoparticles with enhanced photothermal-immunotherapy for ovarian cancer *ACS Nano* **15** 19756–70

[112] Ye P, Li F, Zou J, Luo Y, Wang S, Lu G, Zhang F, Chen C, Long J and Jia R 2022 In situ generation of gold nanoparticles on bacteria-derived magnetosomes for imaging-guided starving/chemodynamic/photothermal synergistic therapy against cancer *Adv. Funct. Mater.* **32** 2110063

[113] Gorgizadeh M, Behzadpour N, Salehi F, Daneshvar F, Vais R D, Nazari-Vanani R, Azarpira N, Lotfi M and Sattarahmady N 2020 A $MnFe_2O_4$/C nanocomposite as a novel theranostic agent in MRI, sonodynamic therapy and photothermal therapy of a melanoma cancer model *J. Alloys Compd.* **816** 152597
[114] Ashkbar A, Rezaei F, Attari F and Ashkevarian S 2020 Treatment of breast cancer *in vivo* by dual photodynamic and photothermal approaches with the aid of curcumin photosensitizer and magnetic nanoparticles *Sci. Rep.* **10** 21206

Sudip Mukherjee, Vijay Sagar Madamsetty, Lipi Pradhan, Anjali Upadhyay and Devyani Yenurkar

Chapter 4

MNPs for cancer diagnosis and imaging

Cancer diagnosis using nanotechnology is a rapidly emerging field that holds great promise for the future of medical care [1–3]. Magnetic nanoparticles (MNPs) are the most promising nanomaterials for use as contrast agents in magnetic resonance imaging (MRI) and induced magnetic hyperthermia. They are also used to improve the sensitivity of biosensors and in various diagnostic tools for cancer treatment. This chapter discusses the use of MNPs in various imaging techniques, the advancement of MRI through the use of MNPs in cancer diagnosis, and the origin of superparamagnetic iron oxide nanoparticles' (SPIONs) unique magnetic properties and their use in cancer diagnosis.

One of nanotechnology's main advantages is its detection of cancer using a noninvasive approach [1, 4, 5]. This advanced method enhances the precision of cancer detection and substantially improves patient comfort and the patient experience [1, 6, 7]. For instance, innovative noninvasive imaging techniques can provide detailed insights into the presence of tumors without the need for painful tissue biopsies [8, 9]. By eliminating this invasive procedure, patients can avoid the physical discomfort and anxiety often associated with traditional diagnostic methods in a patient-focused approach to cancer care [8, 10]. High-sensitivity, noninvasive cancer imaging is crucial for scheduling early treatment [11, 12]. This capability is supported by the unique properties of MNPs, which can significantly enhance imaging quality [13, 14]. Additionally, by making minor modifications to the structure of these nanoparticles, for example, by incorporating a therapeutic agent, it becomes possible to visualize tumor activity and initiate drug delivery simultaneously [14–17]. This innovative approach effectively combines diagnostic imaging with therapeutic intervention, potentially improving patient treatment outcomes [18].

doi:10.1088/978-0-7503-6335-8ch4 © IOP Publishing Ltd 2025. All rights, including for text and data mining (TDM), artificial intelligence (AI) training, and similar technologies, are reserved.

4.1 Overview of cancer diagnosis challenges

Cancer diagnosis involves numerous challenges that can significantly affect the accuracy and speed of identifying the disease [19, 20]. One major challenge is the complexity of symptoms, as many cancers present vague or nonspecific signs that can be mistaken for other conditions [21–23]. This ambiguity often leads to delays in seeking medical attention. Another challenge is the variation in tumor biology among different patients [23]. Tumors can exhibit diverse characteristics, including growth rates, genetic mutations, and responses to treatment [24, 25]. This heterogeneity can complicate the diagnostic process and necessitate advanced and sometimes costly testing [24, 26].

Additionally, the limitations of current diagnostic tools, such as imaging techniques (e.g. x-rays, MRI scans) and biopsies, can hinder early and accurate detection [27–29]. For instance, some tumors may be too small to be detected by imaging or may not provide enough cells for a conclusive biopsy result [30, 31]. Finally, a broad understanding of a patient's medical history, risk factors, and symptoms is critical for an effective diagnosis [32–35]. Health disparities and variations in access to healthcare resources can also pose significant barriers, leading to inequities in cancer diagnosis and treatment across different populations [36]. Addressing these challenges is essential for enhancing diagnostic accuracy, reducing delays, and ultimately improving patient outcomes in cancer care [32, 37, 38]. Here, we will focus on the importance of MNPs as promising imaging tools and discuss how these MNPs can aid in effective early cancer diagnosis.

4.2 Role of magnetic nanoparticles as promising diagnostic tools

MNPs are emerging as promising diagnostic tools in medical and biomedical applications [39, 40]. These tiny particles, with sizes less than 100 nm, possess distinctive magnetic properties that can be utilized for various diagnostic techniques [41]. Their small size allows them to easily circulate in the bloodstream and interact with biological systems at the cellular level. MNPs enhance the sensitivity and specificity of diagnostic imaging methods [42, 43]. Conjugating these nanoparticles using targeting moieties such as peptides or antibodies, which can selectively bind to specific types of tissues or cells, enables the early detection of diseases like cancer [44].

Additionally, MNPs are being used as drug delivery systems, enabling targeted therapies to be accurately delivered to affected areas, thus minimizing side effects [44, 45]. This dual functionality, in which MNPs act as both diagnostic agents and therapeutic carriers, highlights their potential in personalized medicine [46, 47]. Overall, the use of MNPs as diagnostic tools offers a promising avenue for improving disease detection and treatment, paving the way for advancements in healthcare technology [1, 48]. Several techniques, such as MRI, fluorescence, optical, and multimodal methods, use MNPs to help diagnose cancer [42, 49, 50]. In the following section, we will explore the various techniques employed in cancer diagnosis. We will highlight the strengths and applications of each method while also examining the innovative use of MNPs, which have a pronounced ability to enhance the accuracy and efficiency of these diagnostic processes.

4.3 Magnetic resonance imaging

MRI is a sophisticated health imaging procedure that plays a decisive role in diagnosing and evaluating various health conditions [51–53]. It provides high-resolution images of the organs and tissues within the body, enhancing our understanding of patient health and guiding treatment decisions [54, 55].

4.3.1 Mechanism of magnetic nanoparticles in enhancing MRI signals

MNPs help improve the signals produced during MRI [56, 57]. These nanoparticles are designed to influence the magnetic field interactions within the body, enhancing the contrast of images [58]. Altering local magnetic properties increases signal intensity, providing more precise and detailed images of tissues and organs [42, 59]. This enhancement helps in precise diagnosis and beneficial treatment planning in medical imaging applications [42]. MNPs have recently gained substantial interest due to their role as contrast agents in MRI [60]. This interest stems from their unique superparamagnetic properties, particularly at the nanoscale. These properties allow MNPs to improve the visibility of tissues and tumors during imaging [56, 61].

As discussed in previous sections, several key factors influence the effectiveness of MNPs in MRI applications. First, the shape of the nanoparticles can affect how they interact with magnetic fields and biological tissues, impacting their distribution and contrast enhancement [62, 63]. Similarly, the size of the MNPs plays a crucial role; smaller nanoparticles can penetrate biological barriers more efficiently, while larger ones may provide different imaging characteristics [41, 64].

Anisotropy, which refers to the directional dependence of a particle's physical properties, can also significantly influence MNPs' behavior in magnetic fields and their relaxation times in MRI [65]. Magnetization, or the extent to which the nanoparticles can be magnetized, is critical for ensuring strong signals in imaging applications [41, 66]. Finally, the surface chemistry of MNPs is essential for biocompatibility and targeting specific tissues or cells, which can improve the specificity and sensitivity of MRI [67]. Together, these factors dictate the overall performance of MNPs as contrast agents, making them a promising tool in medical imaging. This also highlights recent advancements aimed at improving clinical diagnostics and precision nanomedicine.

4.3.2 Advantages of utilizing nanoparticles for tumor visualization

Nanoparticles represent a groundbreaking advancement in medical imaging, particularly for the visualization of tumors [68]. These nanosized particles possess distinct properties that allow them to infiltrate biological structures and accumulate in tumor tissues more effectively than larger molecules [69]. Their enhanced permeation and retention enable a more evident differentiation between malignant tumors and surrounding healthy tissue during imaging procedures [70]. MNPs can be custom-engineered to deliver specific imaging agents to the target site [71, 72]. By incorporating these agents, nanoparticles significantly improve the contrast and resolution of the images obtained, thus leading to more accurate detection and assessment of tumors. For instance, when these MNPs are combined with techniques such as MRI and computed tomography (CT), they can reveal tumors with exceptional clarity, allowing healthcare professionals to visualize the extent and nature of the disease more precisely [73, 74]. Moreover, MNPs can be designed to target specific biomarkers often overexpressed on the tumor surface. This precision targeting enhances not only the specificity of the imaging process but also the ability to identify different types of tumors based on their unique biological characteristics. By selectively binding to these markers, nanoparticles can provide insights into the tumor's biology and inform treatment decisions [75].

Another significant advantage of nanoparticles is their multifunctional nature. They can be engineered to deliver therapeutic drugs alongside imaging agents, enabling a simultaneous approach to diagnosis and treatment [76, 77]. This capability is particularly promising for developing personalized medicine, where treatments can be tailored based on real-time imaging feedback. Furthermore, the wide range of materials from which nanoparticles can be constructed, such as metals, lipids, and polymers, offers researchers considerable flexibility in designing particles with specific imaging properties [78–81]. This diversity allows nanoparticles to be optimized for various imaging modalities, enhancing their effectiveness across different platforms. Using nanoparticles in tumor visualization enables enhanced imaging capability, targeted accuracy, and potential therapeutic applications. This innovative technology promises to increase our understanding and treatment of cancer, ultimately leading to better patient outcomes and more effective management of this complex disease [82]. In the upcoming sections, we will examine in-depth case studies and illustrative examples highlighting the innovative application of MNPs in MRI. These studies vividly demonstrate how incorporating MNPs into MRI significantly enhances imaging quality and improves contrast, providing clearer and more detailed images. Furthermore, we will explore how these nanoparticles play a crucial role in targeted drug delivery systems, augment diagnostic capabilities, and pave the way for advanced treatment strategies within medical imaging. Through these examples, we aim to illustrate the transformative ability of MNPs to advance patient outcomes and shape the future of medical diagnostics.

4.3.3 Examples of MRI with magnetic nanoparticles

The advantages of magnetic separation processes are that these MNPs can be used to develop rapid, efficient, and lower-cost diagnostic tests while improving sensitivity and specificity [83]. Due to their minimal toxicity and biocompatibility, elevated surface-to-volume ratio, and superparamagnetic properties, iron oxide MNPs are among the most studied MNPs [77]. Iron is exceptionally well tolerated by the human body; thus, the manufacture of iron-based MNPs may be the safest option compared to MNPs based on other elements [82].

Moreover, the efficiency of these MNPs can be further improved by polymer coatings, surface modifications with targeting ligands, etc [84]. The schematic shown in figure 4.1 provides an overview of the various strategies for developing novel MNPs for cancer diagnosis. Polymers such as poly(lactic-co-glycolic acid) (PLGA),

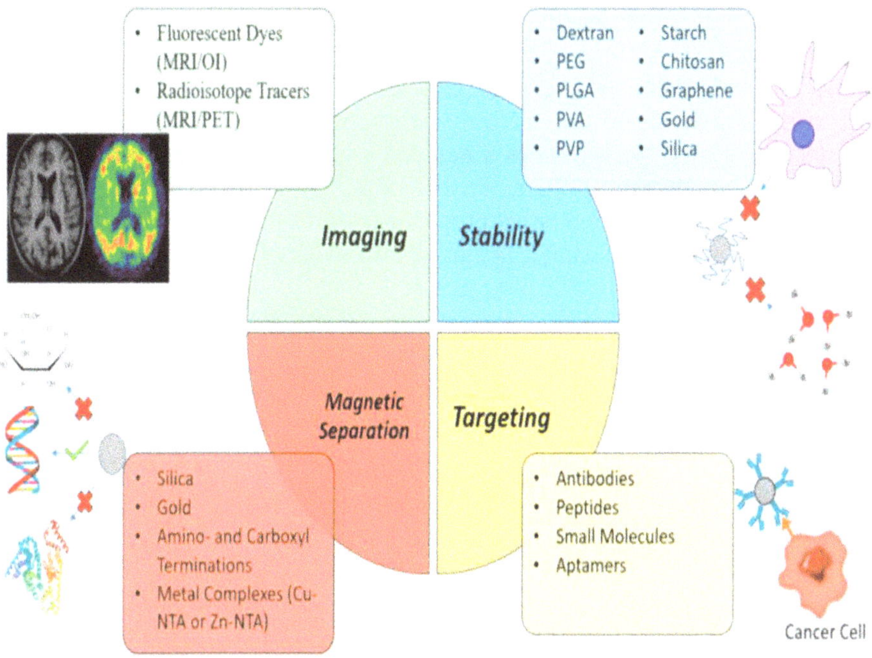

Figure 4.1. Schematic showing the surface modifications and specific applications of MNPs. Adapted from [60]. CC BY 4.0.

polyvinyl alcohol (PVA), polyethylene glycol (PEG), dextran, chitosan, and polyvinylpyrrolidone (PVP) are used to coat MNPs, enhancing their blood circulation time and biocompatibility [60]. Small peptides, aptamers, antibodies, and small-molecule ligands are attached to the surface of MNPs for targeting, further enhancing their selectivity and specificity in cancer imaging [60]. In the following sections, we will discuss the recent advancements in MNPs in MRI imaging.

Recently, scientists developed an effective contrast agent based on SPIONs and compared it with ferucarbotran and ferumoxytol, two conventional contrast agents. The MNPs demonstrated excellent properties *in vitro* and in liver tomography in rats compared to the two conventional contrast agents. Finally, these MNPs showed exceptional safety properties, compelling them to be considered promising candidates for further clinical translation [85].

Chan Ming–Hsien and his team developed a novel approach utilizing kaolinite-modified FePt nanoparticles loaded with the chemotherapeutic agent doxorubicin [86]. This innovative formulation aims to enhance MRI-guided targeted theranostic applications, which combine therapeutic and diagnostic capabilities in cancer treatment [86]. Their study demonstrated promising results, indicating improved targeting and effectiveness of the treatment with minimal side effects. These findings suggest that this targeted delivery system could significantly advance the effectiveness of cancer therapies in clinical applications, demonstrating excellent results [86].

In another study, researchers created an innovative MRI contrast agent specifically designed to target tumors. This agent is based on iron oxide nanoparticles, known as SPIONs, encapsulated within folate-modified chitosan micelle nanoparticles. Chitosan, a biocompatible polymer derived from chitin, enhances the stability and dispersion of the nanoparticles, while folate serves as a targeting moiety, allowing the agent to selectively bind to tumor cells that overexpress folate receptors [87]. Figure 4.2 provides a detailed schematic representation illustrating the synthesis and structural characteristics of MNPs. This study's results showed that these MNPs exhibit impressive properties both *in vitro* (in laboratory settings) and *in vivo* (in living organisms), featuring low levels of cytotoxicity and excellent

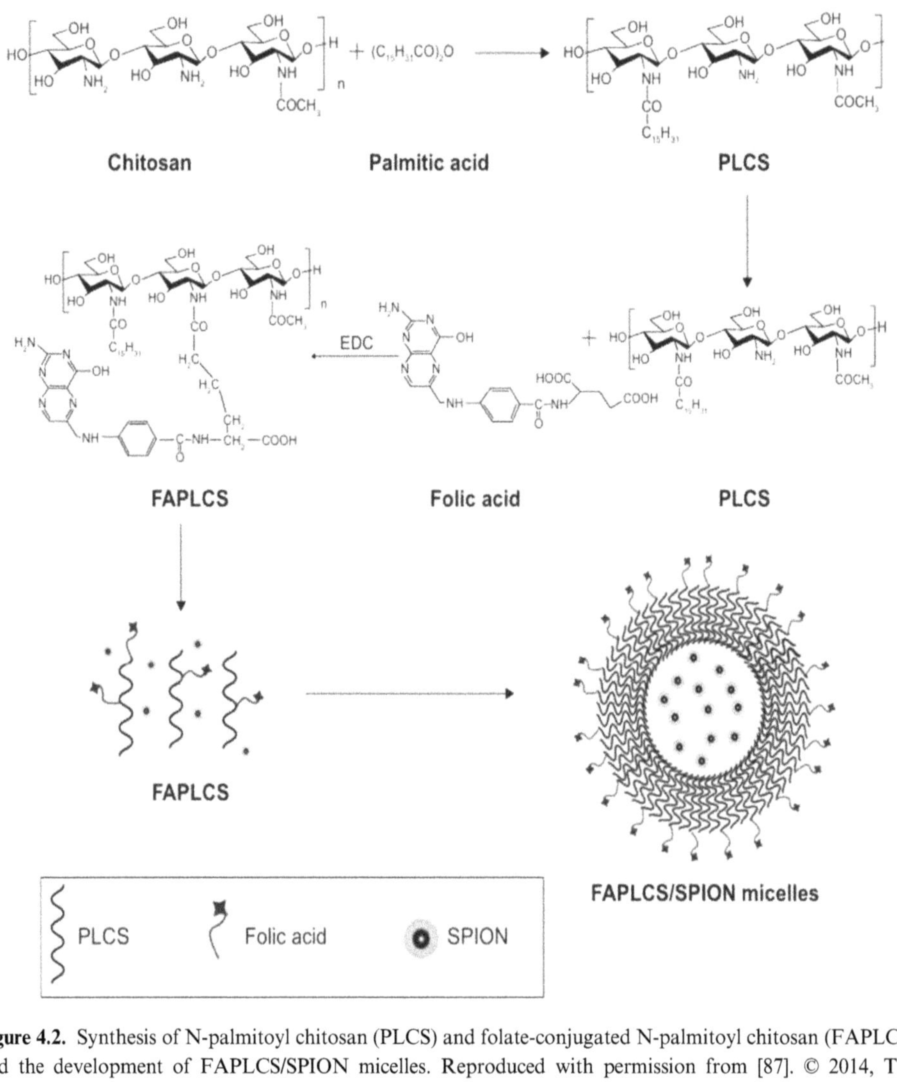

Figure 4.2. Synthesis of N-palmitoyl chitosan (PLCS) and folate-conjugated N-palmitoyl chitosan (FAPLCS) and the development of FAPLCS/SPION micelles. Reproduced with permission from [87]. © 2014, The Author(s), CC BY-NC 3.0. Dove Medical Press Limited reprinted by permission of Informa UK Limited, trading as Taylor & Francis Ltd, https://www.tandfonline.com. Abbreviation: 1-ethyl-3-(3-dimethyl aminopropyl)carbodiimide (eDc), water-soluble carbodiimide usually obtained as the hydrochloride.

biocompatibility. This makes them emerging candidates for increasing the precision and efficacy of MRI in tumor imaging and diagnosis [87].

Xie and colleagues developed a groundbreaking approach that employs lactoferrin-conjugated SPIONs to significantly enhance imaging in MRI applications [88]. Their comprehensive research showed that these novel nanoparticles markedly improve the visualization of glioma cells, a type of brain tumor. This advancement highlights the promising potential of these conjugated nanoparticles in the early diagnosis and ongoing monitoring of brain tumors, which is crucial for effective treatment [88].

The unique design of these SPIONs allows for the precise targeting of glioma cells, thanks to the integration of lactoferrin, a protein known for its ability to bind to specific receptors expressed on cancer cells. This targeted delivery system enhances imaging contrast, enabling clinicians to obtain more transparent, detailed images of tumor regions. As a result, this method may facilitate more accurate diagnosis and improve therapeutic outcomes for patients undergoing treatment for gliomas by enabling more personalized and effective intervention strategies. Overall, this innovative approach represents a significant advancement in MRI technology and its application in neuro-oncology [88].

In a separate study, Gonzalez-Rodriguez and colleagues engineered graphene-conjugated SPIONs to enhance magnetic targeted therapy [89]. This innovative approach involves the integration of graphene, a versatile two-dimensional material, with SPIONs, which are known for their unique magnetic properties. The primary goal of this research was to improve the delivery and efficacy of therapeutic agents. This approach used the magnetic properties of the SPIONs for precise targeting to specific sites within the body, thereby minimizing side effects and maximizing treatment effectiveness [89]. This work represents a significant advancement in nanomedicine, with potential applications in treating various diseases, including cancer.

In a detailed study, Zhang *et al* engineered MNPs coated in methoxy polyethylene glycol (MPEG) and polyethylenimine (PEI) for use as an MRI contrast agent (MPEG-PEI) [90]. The successful coating of SPIONs was confirmed through Fourier transform infrared (FTIR) spectroscopy, revealing that the composition of the particles was approximately 31% PEI and 12% MPEG [90].

Stability experiments indicated that the MPEG-PEI alteration significantly enhanced the stability of MNPs by reducing aggregation. T2 relaxation measurements showed that the R2 values of the MPEG-PEI SPIONs were similar to those of unmodified PEI SPIONs, suggesting that the coating did not compromise their magnetic properties [90]. In T2-weighted MRI tests, MPEG-PEI SPIONs displayed a notable increase in magnetic resonance signal intensity as their concentration in water rose, highlighting their potential as MRI contrast vehicles for improved diagnostic imaging [90].

Ding and his research team successfully developed an innovative nanotheranostic system for MRI-guided combinatorial cancer therapy [91]. The development process of these MNPs is illustrated in detail in figure 4.3, which provides a schematic representation of their formation and functionalization [92]. Upon intravenous injection, these MNPs exhibited a remarkable accumulation in tumor tissues, a

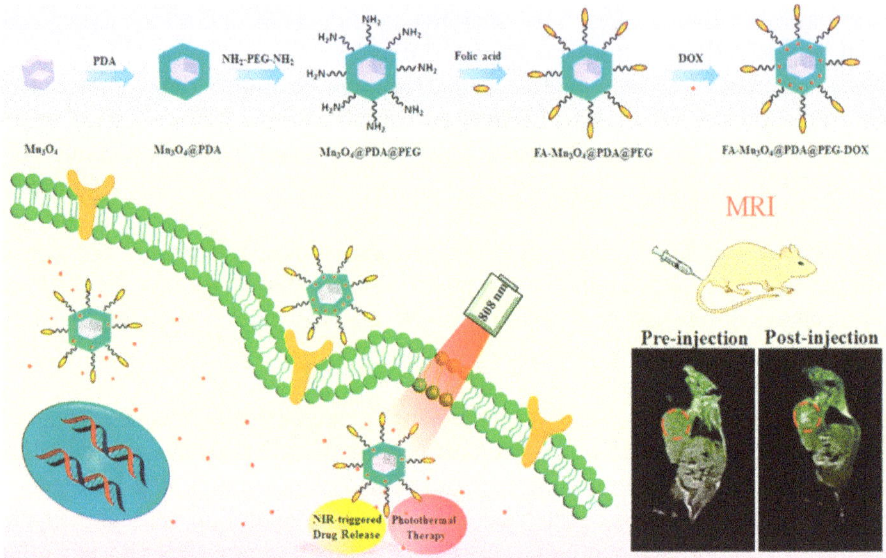

Figure 4.3. Schematic representation depicting the design and synthesis of core–shell synergetic nano-theranostic nanoparticles (Mn_3O_4 coated with polydopamine (PDA), Mn_3O_4@PDA) used for chemo-photothermal therapy. Adapted with permission from [92]. CC BY 4.0.

finding demonstrated through MRI imaging techniques [91]. This targeted accumulation is crucial for enhancing the efficiency of cancer therapy while minimizing toxicity to healthy tissues [92].

These MNPs possessed several advantageous properties, including highly favorable magnetic characteristics that facilitated imaging and targeted therapy [92]. Additionally, they demonstrated good biocompatibility, meaning they were well tolerated by the body and did not provoke significant adverse reactions. Most importantly, the toxicity profile of these nanoparticles was significantly improved compared to traditional Gd(III)-based nanosystems. This enhanced safety profile suggests that paramagnetic manganese (Mn) ions can provide substantial benefits in developing the next generation of theranostic contrast agents, positioning them as a promising alternative in cancer diagnostics and treatment [92].

4.4 Fluorescence imaging

Fluorescence imaging is a medical imaging technique that utilizes the fluorescence properties of specific molecules to detect and visualize cancerous tissues [93–95]. This method introduces specific fluorescent dyes or probes into the body, which bind to cancer cells [93]. When exposed to a light source, these dyes emit fluorescent light, differentiating healthy and cancerous tissues [94]. This technique is valuable in cancer detection, as it enhances the visibility of tumors during surgical procedures or imaging studies, enabling clinicians to make more accurate diagnoses and treatment decisions [95]. Fluorescence imaging can also provide real-time information about a tumor's characteristics, improving the overall management of cancer patients.

4.4.1 Principles of fluorescence in cancer detection

Fluorescence is a revolutionary technique in the fight against cancer, transforming the way in which diagnoses are made. At its core, fluorescence relies on the ability of specific molecules to absorb light and subsequently emit it at different wavelengths [96]. This dynamic process starts when a fluorescent probe is excited by a specific light source. As these probes absorb energy, they enter an excited state, quickly releasing that energy as light as they revert to their original state [97]. This emitted fluorescence can be detected, offering crucial insights into the presence of cancerous cells with remarkable sensitivity. In cancer detection, specially designed fluorescent markers can effectively target and bind to cancer cells, allowing for precise imaging and visualization. For instance, fluorescent dyes linked to antibodies recognizing tumor-specific proteins increase the visibility of tumors in advanced imaging systems, including fluorescence microscopy or endoscopy, leading to earlier and more accurate diagnoses [98].

The application of fluorescence extends beyond imaging; it is also essential in flow cytometry. Here, cells stained with fluorescent markers are analyzed as they pass through a laser beam, permitting detailed quantification and characterization of cell populations [99]. This is particularly invaluable for diagnosing blood cancers and monitoring treatment effectiveness. Recent technological advancements have further amplified the capabilities of fluorescence-based methods, paving the way for fluorescence lifetime imaging and multiplex assays. These innovations permit the simultaneous detection of multiple targets, providing a richer and more nuanced understanding of tumor dynamics. In essence, the principles of fluorescence not only equip healthcare professionals with enhanced methods for detecting and diagnosing cancer but also offer hope for improving patient outcomes and advancing cancer research in unprecedented ways [99].

Figure 4.4 illustrates the use of fluorescence detectors in cancer therapy, highlighting the role of various fluorescent agents employed in this setting [98]. These fluorescent agents are instrumental in several key applications, including cancer detection at an early stage, tumor type characterization, and targeted therapy of cancerous cells. The detection process allows the identification of malignant tissues, while the characterization capability helps to determine the stage and type of cancer, allowing tailored therapy plans to be developed. Furthermore, fluorescence-based therapies utilize these agents to target and treat cancer cells selectively, improving the treatment's effectiveness while minimizing damage to surrounding healthy tissues [98].

4.4.2 Integration of magnetic nanoparticles for targeted fluorescence

The integration of MNPs plays a crucial role in enhancing targeted fluorescence for cancer detection [44]. By leveraging the unique properties of these nanoparticles, we can achieve precise localization of cancerous cells. This method involves attaching specific fluorescent markers to MNPs, allowing for improved visualization by fluorescence imaging techniques. As a result, medical professionals can detect

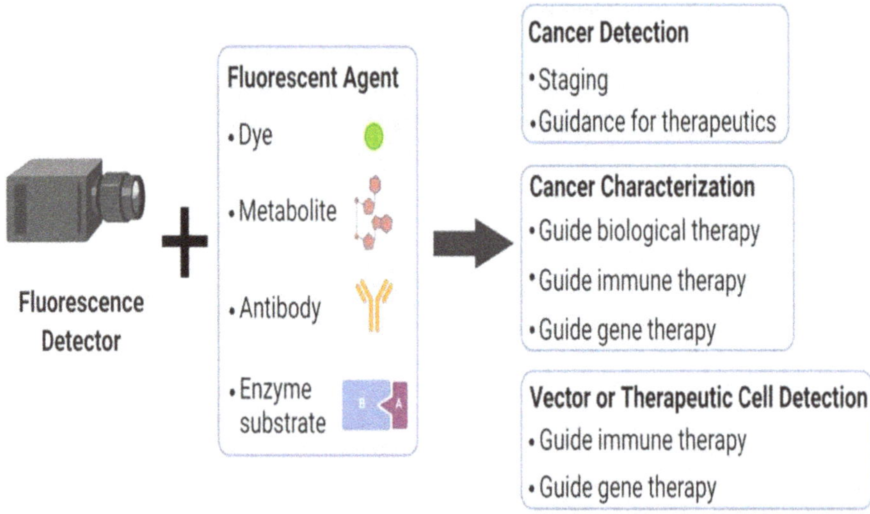

Figure 4.4. Schematic illustration depicting the application of fluorescence detectors in cancer therapy and the fluorescent agents used in this application. Adapted from [98], Copyright (2021), with permission from Elsevier.

tumors early and plan appropriate treatment options, which results in better patient outcomes [44, 75].

The advantages of enhanced sensitivity and specificity in tumor identification through fluorescence techniques are crucial for advancing cancer diagnosis and treatment [11]. Enhanced sensitivity allows clinicians to detect tiny clusters of tumor cells or precancerous lesions that traditional imaging methods might miss. This early detection is vital, as it can lead to timely interventions that may improve a patient's prognosis and survival rates. On the other hand, increasing specificity ensures that the signals detected are accurately associated with tumor presence, thereby reducing the occurrence of false positives. This reliability is essential for minimizing unnecessary anxiety for patients and avoiding unwarranted tests or treatments that can arise from misdiagnosis [11, 100].

Moreover, these improvements in sensitivity and specificity can facilitate more precise and targeted therapies. A clearer understanding of the tumor's characteristics helps healthcare workers to design personalized treatment plans customized to a patient's unique cancer profile [101]. Overall, integrating advanced fluorescence techniques can significantly transform the oncology environment, enabling more effective strategies for cancer management and improving overall patient care [100].

4.4.3 Examples of fluorescence imaging with magnetic nanoparticles

In the following sections, we will explore recent advancements in fluorescence imaging techniques that utilize MNPs. These innovative methods enhance clarity and accuracy in biomedical research, allowing us to observe biological processes and structures in greater detail. We will provide examples that illustrate how these techniques improve our understanding of complex biological systems and contribute to advancements in medical science. These sophisticated methods take advantage of MNPs' unique properties and can easily be controlled using external magnetic fields. This capability enables targeted imaging of specific tissues or cells. As a result, this approach enhances the detection of fluorescent signals, making it an invaluable tool for studying biological processes, tracking drug delivery, and diagnosing diseases at the molecular level.

Researchers have innovatively developed two types of conjugated polymers: cationic polymers that emit a striking blue fluorescence and anionic polymers that glow in vibrant green [102]. These polymers are dual-color fluorescence probes, allowing for advanced imaging techniques. They are anchored to the surfaces of negatively charged MNPs through a carefully controlled process of sequential electrostatic adsorption, which ensures a strong attachment (figure 4.5) [102]. These conjugated polymers are notable for their impressive properties, including significant extinction coefficients that enhance their fluorescence and high quantum yields of 82% for the blue-emissive PFN and 62% for the green-emissive ThPFS. When these specially crafted nanoparticles are introduced into cellular environments, they exhibit remarkable cellular uptake while maintaining low toxicity levels, making them safe for biological applications. This combination of qualities renders them exceptionally suitable for simultaneous noninvasive MRI and fluorescence imaging, paving the way for medical diagnostics and research advancements [102].

In recent years, the development of specific magneto-fluorescent nanoparticles has attracted considerable interest within the scientific community. These unique nanoparticles combine magnetic and fluorescent properties, making them highly valuable for various applications, including targeted drug delivery, medical imaging, and biosensors. Researchers are particularly focused on optimizing their synthesis and functionalization to enhance their stability, biocompatibility, and efficacy in different biological environments [41, 103]. This growing interest reflects the

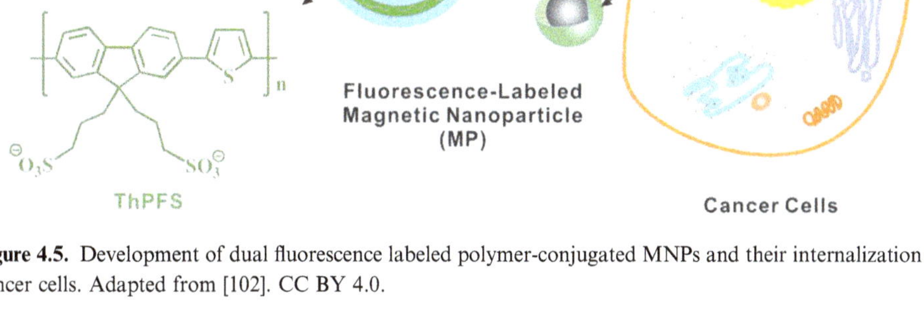

Figure 4.5. Development of dual fluorescence labeled polymer-conjugated MNPs and their internalization by cancer cells. Adapted from [102]. CC BY 4.0.

potential of magneto-fluorescent nanoparticles to revolutionize fields such as nanomedicine and diagnostics.

Scientists have developed a self-assembled chitosan nanocomposite, Chit-IOCO NPs, which combines cerium oxide with SPIONs [103]. This theranostic approach contains a Cy5 dye and methotrexate (MTX), acting as an anticancer agent while providing negative contrast for MRI imaging. *In vivo* studies showed that Chit-IOCO-Cy5-MTX improved tumor uptake and retention compared to nanoceria without MTX. Safety assessments in mice revealed no major differences between the treatment and control groups [103]. In a recent study, scientists developed SPIONs functionalized through a CXCR4 receptor binding ligand [104]. The composition of these SPIONs was confirmed using transmission electron microscopy (TEM) and x-ray diffraction (XRD). Fluorescently loaded SPIONs improved imaging contrast in Jurkat cancer cells, and flow cytometry revealed effective blocking of CXCR4 receptors. These results highlight the potential of SPIONs in targeted cancer therapy and advanced cancer diagnostics [104].

In a further study, scientists developed a magnetic micromesh combined with fluorescent MNPs to enhance cancer targeting [105]. This technique allows for the magnetic targeting of individual fluorescent metal nanoshells (FMNs). Real-time fluorescence intravital microscopy images demonstrated that these MNPs were preserved in the tumor blood vessels and immediately nearby tissues. Additionally, this magnetically enhanced targeting improved the biological activity of molecules linked to the nanoparticles [105]. A recent article highlighted the development of Fe_3O_4/graphene nanosystems for multimodal imaging and cancer therapy. The review covers structural features, imaging performance, toxicity, efficiency, and the ability to ablate cancer cells using therapeutic approaches [106].

4.5 Optical imaging techniques

Optical imaging techniques are methods used to capture images by utilizing visible light and other forms of electromagnetic radiation [107]. These techniques have diverse roles in various subjects, including materials science, biology, and medicine, as they allow for the visualization of structures and processes at both the macro and micro levels [107]. Standard methods include techniques such as fluorescence microscopy, optical coherence tomography, and confocal microscopy, each offering unique advantages for observing specimens in real time and with high resolution. Researchers and clinicians can gain deeper insights into the composition, function, and dynamics of biological and physical systems through these methods.

4.5.1 Challenges and limitations in optical applications

Thorough examination and resolution of the challenges and limitations associated with optical applications in cancer detection are crucial for advancing this field. Several key factors must be addressed to enhance the efficacy of these technologies [108].

First, the sensitivity and specificity of optical techniques are paramount. Sensitivity refers to the ability to correctly identify cancerous tissues, while specificity pertains to the ability to distinguish between cancerous and non-cancerous tissues. Improving these metrics is essential for reducing false positives and false negatives, which can lead to misdiagnoses and inappropriate treatment plans. Second, the optical properties of different types of tissues are notably variable. Factors such as tissue type, hydration levels, and underlying pathologies can significantly affect optical signal interpretation. Understanding and accounting for this variability is necessary to develop more reliable optical diagnostic methods [108, 109].

Moreover, the development of robust imaging systems is vital. These systems must be designed to produce clear and actionable data under various conditions. This requires advancements in imaging technology, as well as ensuring that these systems can be integrated effectively into clinical workflows and manage the complexities of real-world medical environments. In addition, there is a pressing need for standardized protocols for numerous optical modalities. Establishing these protocols will ensure that tests can be performed consistently across different laboratories and clinical settings, which is essential for obtaining reliable and comparable results [110].

Addressing these challenges is critical for enhancing the overall effectiveness of optical technologies in cancer diagnosis. Improving accuracy and reliability can ultimately contribute to better patient outcomes, facilitating earlier intervention and potentially more effective treatment strategies for cancer patients.

4.5.2 Application of magnetic nanoparticles to improve optical contrast

The application of MNPs plays a vital role in enhancing optical contrast, making them a valuable tool in various scientific and medical fields. These nanometer-sized particles have unique magnetic and optical properties, which are coupled to improve image quality. When incorporated into imaging techniques, MNPs interact with light to increase the visibility of specific structures or tissues, leading to sharper and more detailed images [76].

In medical imaging, for example, these nanoparticles can be strategically targeted to specific cells or tissues, enabling radiologists to distinguish between healthy and diseased areas more effectively. By increasing the contrast between different types of tissues, MNPs facilitate earlier detection of conditions such as tumors or other abnormalities. This innovative approach enhances diagnostic accuracy and holds great promise for developing more effective treatment strategies [75].

4.5.3 Examples of the use of magnetic nanoparticles to improve optical contrast in cancer detection

In a study, scientists exploited dye-based MNPs with near-infrared optical imaging properties. The biodistribution and tumor localization of these MNPs were evaluated in mice with xenograft breast tumors, both with and without an external magnetic field. The MNPs comprised an iron oxide magnetic core covered with oleic acid (OA) and stabilized using an amphiphilic block copolymer [75].

At 48 h post-administration, the MNPs gradually localized within the tumor and showed a slow decline for 11 days. Furthermore, after one hour of magnetic field exposure directed at the tumor, the localization of MNPs in the tumor was significantly enhanced. These MNPs can be further exploited for combined multi-modal imaging and drug delivery, improving cancer identification, providing sustained treatment, and enabling ongoing monitoring of tumor therapeutic impacts over time [75].

Another report by Yan *et al* discussed the surface fabrication of SPIONs with the Cy5.5-labeled peptide GX1, a marker associated with angiogenesis in gastric cancer [111]. *In vivo* optical imaging showed that the targeted probe accumulated primarily in the tumors. Additionally, it generated dark distinguishing spots at the tumor site in MRI images [111].

4.6 Multimodal imaging methods

Multimodal imaging methods for cancer detection involve various imaging technologies that work together to improve the accuracy and effectiveness of cancerous lesion identification [112]. By combining techniques such as MRI, CT, PET, and ultrasound, healthcare professionals can obtain a comprehensive view of the body's internal structures. This integrated approach enhances early detection, facilitates better diagnosis, and allows for more precise treatment planning, ultimately leading to improved patient outcomes in the battle against cancer [112].

Figure 4.6 provides a detailed overview of various multimodal imaging systems, including MRI, fluorescence imaging, CT, positron emission tomography (PET),

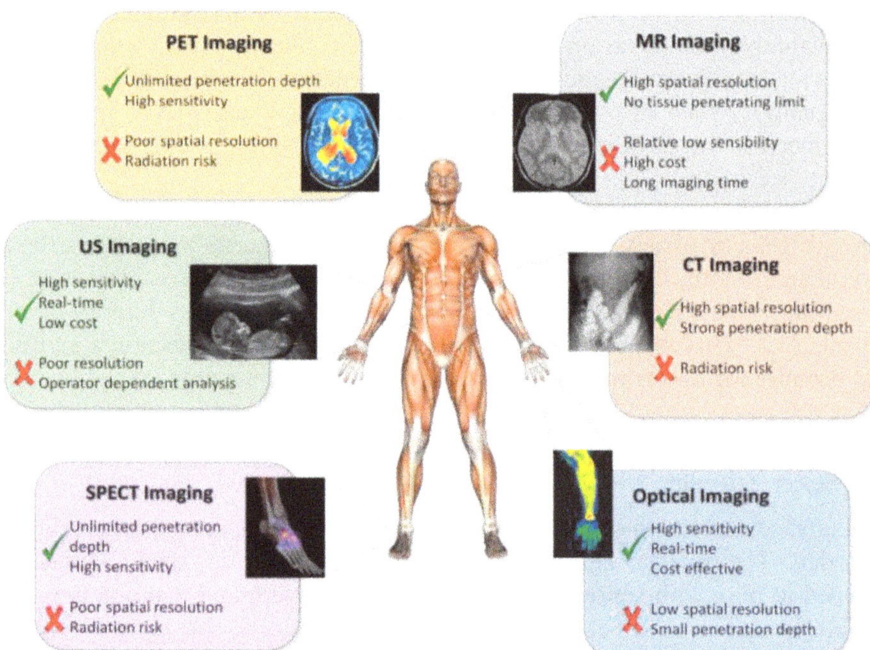

Figure 4.6. Schematic representation of different imaging modalities used in multimodal imaging. Adapted from [112]. CC BY 4.0.

and optical imaging methods [112]. It discusses each method's advantages and disadvantages, highlighting their distinct physical principles and operational characteristics. Additionally, the figure explores the applications of multimodal molecular imaging, specifically in cancer research, emphasizing how hybrid MNPs enhance imaging capabilities and improve diagnostic accuracy. This comprehensive analysis aims to clarify the strengths and limitations of each imaging modality in oncological research and clinical practice [112].

4.6.1 Definition and importance of multimodal imaging

Multimodal approaches use multiple methods or modes of communication and instruction to enhance understanding and learning. These approaches are significant because they accommodate different learning styles and preferences, allowing for a more inclusive and effective educational experience. By incorporating various modalities, such as visual, auditory, and kinesthetic elements, multimodal approaches can engage learners more profoundly and facilitate better retention of information [113].

Multimodal imaging integrates multiple imaging techniques to provide a comprehensive understanding of a subject, particularly in medical diagnostics and research. This innovative approach combines various modalities, such as MRI, CT, PET, and ultrasound. Each imaging technique offers unique information about anatomical structures, physiological functions, and metabolic processes, enabling clinicians and researchers to see a complete picture of a patient's health [113, 114].

The main benefit of multimodal imaging is its ability to provide detailed and complementary insights that single-modality imaging might miss. For instance, while MRI is excellent for visualizing soft tissue structures, CT scans are particularly effective in assessing bone integrity and detecting bleeding or tumors. By combining these modalities, healthcare providers can achieve superior diagnostic accuracy, which is crucial for developing effective treatment strategies [114].

Moreover, multimodal imaging plays a significant role in personalized medicine. It allows healthcare practitioners to design treatment plans. For example, integrating PET scans with CT in oncology can help accurately stage tumors, monitor treatment response, and assess recurrence [115].

In summary, multimodal imaging enhances diagnostic precision, guides treatment decisions, and improves patient outcomes. Its interdisciplinary applications make it a valuable clinical practice and research tool, bridging the gap between various imaging technologies to foster a more holistic approach to patient care.

4.6.2 Synergistic effects of combining MRI, fluorescence, and optical imaging

The synergistic effects obtained by integrating MRI, optical, and fluorescence imaging significantly enhance diagnostic and therapeutic capabilities [116]. By combining these advanced imaging modalities, researchers and clinicians can better visualize biological processes and structures more comprehensively. MRI provides detailed anatomical information with excellent spatial resolution, while fluorescence imaging allows for the visualization of specific biomolecules and cellular processes in real time, leveraging the unique properties of fluorescent markers. Optical imaging further enhances this understanding by offering high-resolution tissue architecture and dynamic images. Together, these techniques can improve the accuracy of disease detection, facilitate targeted therapies, and enable better monitoring of treatment responses, ultimately leading to more personalized and effective patient care [117].

4.6.3 Examples of multimodal systems incorporating magnetic nanoparticles

Examples of multimodal systems that incorporate MNPs include advanced drug delivery systems, where these nanoparticles facilitate targeted treatment by delivering medications directly to specific cells or tissues [56]. Additionally, they are utilized in diagnostic imaging techniques, enhancing the contrast in imaging modalities such as MRI and providing real-time monitoring of biological processes. Other applications use MNPs in cancer therapy, as they can be employed for hyperthermic treatment. This generates localized heat in tumors through the switching of magnetic fields [118].

Various published review articles have outlined the latest improvements in multimodal imaging systems, explicitly focusing on MNPs and their theranostic applications in cancer treatment [18, 119]. Other reviews have discussed the physicochemical properties of these MNPs and compared various synthesis methods for MNPs, including SPIONs, used in the development of multimodal contrast agents [120, 121].

Scientists successfully created multifunctional magnetic-Ni-doped fluorescent $ZnAl_2O_4$ NPs [122], which displayed fluorescence in the second biological near-infrared window. This innovative development holds tremendous promise for advancing biomedical functions [122]. Hu *et al* successfully developed a dual-modal nanoprobe for tumor imaging that combined magnetic and fluorescent properties [123]. This advanced probe was synthesized from a unique star-like polymer structure that enhanced its efficacy. During *in vivo* MRI studies, the nanoprobe significantly improved the visualization of tumor boundaries, allowing for precise delineation. Furthermore, it exhibited remarkable tumor-targeting capabilities, with fluorescence intensity peaking within the tumor, representing an exceptional development in tumor recognition and examination [123].

Dual-modality probes offer a versatile approach for studying diseases at different dimensions. Scientists created a collection of MRI/FI nanoprobes using three main processes: (i) adsorbing dialkylcarbocyanine dyes on MNPs, (ii) coating MNPs with phospholipids, and (iii) functionalizing MNPs with targeting ligands via bioconjugation [124]. The DiI (1,1'-dioctadecyl-3,3,3',3'-tetramethylindocarbocyanine perchlorate)/DiR (1,1'-dioctadecyl-3,3,3',3'-tetramethylindotricarbocyanine iodide)/MNP nanoprobes offered stability and superior indication contrast in MRI scans and near-infrared fluorescence imaging, showing promise for tumor diagnostics, intraoperative imaging, and biopsies. This approach facilitates the design of effective multimodal imaging probes [124]. In subsequent groundbreaking research, scientists innovatively combined MRI with fluorescence imaging utilizing MNPs, enabling an advanced assessment of cancer at multiple spatial scales and resolutions. Figure 4.7 shows an MRI probe developed using Fe_3O_4 nanoparticles. This fluorescence probe

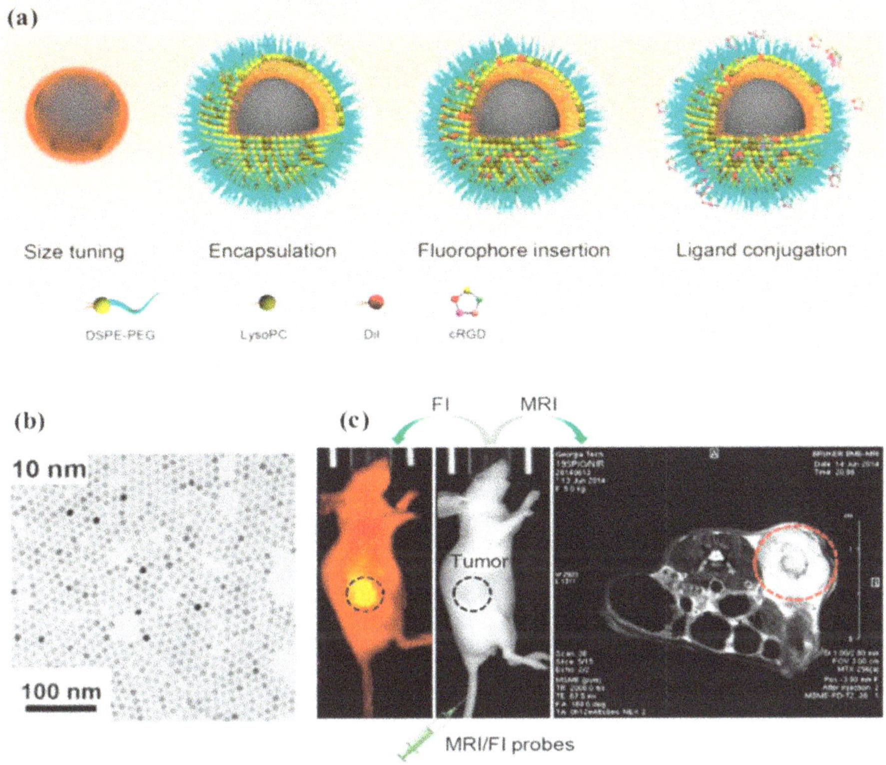

Figure 4.7. (a) Schematic diagram of MRI/FI nanoprobes developed using MNPs, lipid PEG, fluorescent dye, and targeting ligands. (b) TEM image of the Fe_3O_4 NPs, and (c) the use of MRI/fluorescent nanoprobes to produce images of tumor-bearing mice. Parts (a) and (b) adapted from [59]. CC BY 4.0. Part (c) adapted with permission from [125]. Copyright (2020) American Chemical Society.

was synthesized via the physical adsorption of dialkylcarbocyanine dyes on the Fe_3O_4 nanoparticles [59]. Additionally, the surface of these MNPs was modified by conjugating a targeting ligand, which further enhanced the contrast delivery efficiency in MRI and fluorescence imaging [59]. This powerful approach offers a clearer understanding of the disease, enhancing diagnostic capabilities and paving the way for more efficient treatments. These agents play a crucial role in enhancing the clarity and sensitivity of the images produced, allowing healthcare professionals to obtain a more detailed view of internal structures.

By improving the quality of the images, contrast agents facilitate more accurate diagnoses, which are essential for effective patient care and treatment planning [59, 124].

Researchers created a groundbreaking multifunctional nanoagent called vortex nanoring Fe_3O_4 (VNFG) [126]. This unique nanoagent consisted of a ring-like vortex-domain iron oxide core, which provides magnetic properties, and a shell composed of gadolinium oxide, enhancing its imaging capabilities. VNFG was specifically designed to support dual-modality MRI, enabling more precise visualization of tumors. Its innovative structure was also intended for application in guided magnetic thermal cancer therapy, providing a promising approach to more effective cancer treatment [126]. Xue *et al* successfully developed an innovative delivery system utilizing macrophages to enhance the transport of Fe@Fe_3O_4-DHCA nanoparticles, which were 14 nm in size [127]. This approach significantly improved the effectiveness of MRI and magnetic hyperthermia in the treatment of solid tumors [127]. Another study designed a representative trimodal CT/OFI/MRI nanoprobe, as depicted in figure 4.8 [128]. The core was made from a Cy5 mesoporous silica shell covered in iodinated oil, which functioned as a CT contrast agent [128]. This nanoprobe was surface-altered with PEG to improve its bioavailability and extend its circulation time in the bloodstream [128].

Many trimodal probes that combine optical fluorescence imaging (OFI), MRI, and CT have been primarily pursued to comprehensively diagnose, visualize, and delineate cancerous tissues and tumors [18, 129, 130]. These innovative diagnostic devices are characterized by their multifaceted compositions, which stem from the intricate interplay of various contrast agents used in OFI, MRI, and CT modalities. Each of these imaging techniques contributes unique advantages to tumor assessment: OFI offers high-resolution imaging at the cellular level through fluorescent

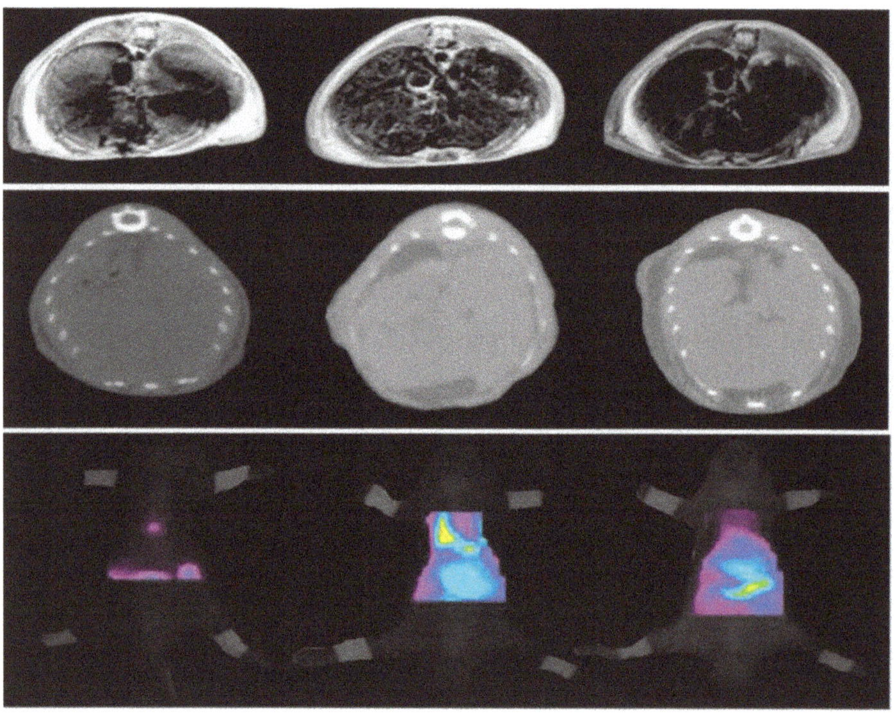

Figure 4.8. Trimodal CT/OFI/MRI nanoprobe use for *in vivo* imaging. T2-weighted MR (top row), CT (middle row), and fluorescence images (third row) of mouse livers after intravenous infusion of trimodal MNPs. Reproduced with permission from [128]. © 2013, The Author(s), CC BY-NC 3.0. Dove Medical Press Limited reprinted by permission of Informa UK Limited, trading as Taylor & Francis Ltd, http://www.tandfonline.com.

markers that highlight specific biological processes; MRI provides detailed anatomical information and tissue characterization using powerful magnetic fields; and CT delivers rapid cross-sectional images that enable thorough examination of the tumor's size, shape, and location [5, 129–131].

The complexity of these probes arises from the need to optimize the effectiveness of each imaging modality while ensuring the compatibility of the different contrast agents involved. In select studies, researchers have also begun to investigate the incorporation of additional therapeutic functions within these trimodal systems. This innovative approach aims to diagnose and visualize tumors and enable real-time treatment, thereby enhancing the overall efficacy of cancer management strategies [131–134].

4.7 Summary of the benefits of using magnetic nanoparticles in cancer diagnosis

MNPs present a range of significant benefits in cancer diagnosis. One of their primary advantages is their capability to enhance imaging techniques. MNPs can be utilized as contrast agents in MRI, where their magnetic properties enhance the contrast and resolution of images. This enhanced imaging allows for more precise detection of tumors, enabling healthcare professionals to identify cancerous cells at earlier stages. Moreover, MNPs can be engineered to target specific types of cancer cells. Due to their small size and surface modifications, these nanoparticles can be designed to bind to particular biomarkers associated with tumors. This targeted approach improves the accuracy of diagnoses and minimizes the impact on surrounding healthy tissues. As a result, the likelihood of obtaining false positives or negatives is reduced, allowing for more reliable clinical assessments.

Additionally, the magnetic properties of these nanoparticles facilitate their easy manipulation. They can be directed to selected areas of the body by applying external magnetic fields, enhancing the precision of their delivery. This targeted delivery system can also be used for drug delivery in therapeutics. However, in the context of diagnostics, it helps to concentrate imaging agents at tumor sites, further improving detection capabilities. Furthermore, MNPs are biocompatible and can be designed to degrade safely within the body after their diagnostic role is complete, reducing potential side effects and making them a safer option for patients. Their versatility also allows for the combination of imaging and therapeutic functions, paving the way for innovative approaches such as theranostics, which integrates therapy and diagnostics in a single platform. In conclusion, using MNPs in cancer diagnosis enhances the accuracy and effectiveness of imaging techniques, allows for targeted delivery to cancer cells, and contributes to improved patient safety, making MNPs a valuable asset in modern oncology.

4.7.1 Future perspectives and potential developments of magnetic nanoparticles in diagnosis and imaging

The field of MNPs has emerged as a promising area of research for enhancing diagnostic and imaging techniques in medicine. Future perspectives and potential developments in the use of MNPs for diagnosis and imaging warrant further investigation. Due to their exceptional biocompatibility and magnetic properties, these nanoparticles can potentially transform the way in which we detect and visualize various diseases. Future prospects in this field include the development of novel MNP formulations that can improve the specificity and sensitivity of imaging modalities. Additionally, there is growing interest in optimizing the surface coatings of these particles to facilitate targeted drug delivery and improve imaging contrast. Further advancements may focus on integrating MNPs with other cutting-edge technologies, such as biosensors and molecular imaging agents, to provide real-time monitoring of disease progression at the molecular level. Researchers are also investigating the use of MNPs in nanomedicine, where they could play a crucial role in therapeutic interventions, enabling simultaneous diagnosis and treatment. In summary, the potential developments in the use of MNPs for diagnosis and imaging are vast, as they could lead to promising innovations that revolutionize medical diagnostics, enhance patient outcomes, and ultimately pave the way for more personalized treatment approaches.

References and further reading

[1] Al-Thani A N, Jan A G, Abbas M, Geetha M and Sadasivuni K K 2024 Nanoparticles in cancer theragnostic and drug delivery: a comprehensive review *Life Sci.* **352** 122899

[2] Lankoff A M, Czerwińska M and Kruszewski M 2024 Advances in nanotheranostic systems for concurrent cancer imaging and therapy: an overview of the last 5 years *Molecules* **29** 5985

[3] Alromi D A, Madani S Y and Seifalian A 2021 Emerging application of magnetic nanoparticles for diagnosis and treatment of cancer *Polymers* **13** 4146

[4] Peixoto L, Magalhães R, Navas D, Moraes S, Redondo C, Morales R, Araújo J P and Sousa C T 2020 Magnetic nanostructures for emerging biomedical applications *Appl. Phys. Rev.* **7** 011310

[5] Li X, Li W, Wang M and Liao Z 2021 Magnetic nanoparticles for cancer theranostics: advances and prospects *J. Control. Release* **335** 437–48

[6] Ganguly S and Margel S 2023 Bioimaging probes based on magneto-fluorescent nanoparticles *Pharmaceutics* **15** 686

[7] Crosby D, Bhatia S, Brindle K M, Coussens L M, Dive C, Emberton M, Esener S, Fitzgerald R C, Gambhir S S and Kuhn P 2022 Early detection of cancer *Science* **375** eaay9040

[8] Shahalaei M, Azad A K, Sulaiman W M A W, Derakhshani A, Mofakham E B, Mallandrich M, Kumarasamy V and Subramaniyan V 2024 A review of metallic nanoparticles: present issues and prospects focused on the preparation methods, characterization techniques, and their theranostic applications *Front. Chem.* **12** 1398979

[9] Dhiman A, Rana D, Benival D and Garkhal K 2024 Comprehensive insights into glioblastoma multiforme: drug delivery challenges and multimodal treatment strategies *Ther. Deliv.* **16** 87–115

[10] Sahu S C 2024 *Nanomaterials in Medicine: Applications and Challenges* (Bhopal: AG Publishing House)

[11] Fitzgerald R C, Antoniou A C, Fruk L and Rosenfeld N 2022 The future of early cancer detection *Nat. Med.* **28** 666–77
[12] Cheng Z, Ma J, Yin L, Yu L, Yuan Z, Zhang B, Tian J and Du Y 2023 Non-invasive molecular imaging for precision diagnosis of metastatic lymph nodes: opportunities from preclinical to clinical applications *Eur. J. Nucl. Med. Mol. Imaging* **50** 1111–33
[13] Anik M I, Hossain M K, Hossain I, Mahfuz A, Rahman M T and Ahmed I 2021 Recent progress of magnetic nanoparticles in biomedical applications: a review *Nano Select* **2** 1146–86
[14] Zhao S, Yu X, Qian Y, Chen W and Shen J 2020 Multifunctional magnetic iron oxide nanoparticles: an advanced platform for cancer theranostics *Theranostics* **10** 6278
[15] Manzari M T, Shamay Y, Kiguchi H, Rosen N, Scaltriti M and Heller D A 2021 Targeted drug delivery strategies for precision medicines *Nat. Rev. Mater.* **6** 351–70
[16] Izci M, Maksoudian C, Manshian B B and Soenen S J 2021 The use of alternative strategies for enhanced nanoparticle delivery to solid tumors *Chem. Rev.* **121** 1746–803
[17] Vikal A, Maurya R, Patel P, Paliwal S R, Narang R K, Gupta G D and Kurmi B D 2024 Exploring metal-organic frameworks (MOFs) in drug delivery: a concise overview of synthesis approaches, versatile applications, and current challenges *Appl. Mater. Today* **41** 102443
[18] Zhao J, Chen J, Ma S, Liu Q, Huang L, Chen X, Lou K and Wang W 2018 Recent developments in multimodality fluorescence imaging probes *Acta Pharm. Sin.* B **8** 320–38
[19] Wu L and Qu X 2015 Cancer biomarker detection: recent achievements and challenges *Chem. Soc. Rev.* **44** 2963–97
[20] Rasheed S, Kanwal T, Ahmad N, Fatima B, Najam-ul-Haq M and Hussain D 2024 Advances and challenges in portable optical biosensors for onsite detection and point-of-care diagnostics *TrAC, Trends Anal. Chem.* **173** 117640
[21] Damhus C S, Risør M B, Brodersen J B and Jønsson A B R 2024 Rethinking the logic of early diagnosis in cancer *Health* **29** 3–22
[22] Renzi C, Kaushal A, Emery J, Hamilton W, Neal R D, Rachet B, Rubin G, Singh H, Walter F M and de Wit N J 2019 Comorbid chronic diseases and cancer diagnosis: disease-specific effects and underlying mechanisms *Nat. Rev. Clin. Oncol.* **16** 746–61
[23] Bi W L, Hosny A, Schabath M B, Giger M L, Birkbak N J, Mehrtash A, Allison T, Arnaout O, Abbosh C and Dunn I F 2019 Artificial intelligence in cancer imaging: clinical challenges and applications *CA: Cancer J. Clin.* **69** 127–57
[24] Dagogo-Jack I and Shaw A T 2018 Tumour heterogeneity and resistance to cancer therapies *Nat. Rev. Clin. Oncol.* **15** 81–94
[25] Liu B, Zhou H, Tan L, Siu K T H and Guan X-Y 2024 Exploring treatment options in cancer: tumor treatment strategies *Signal Transduct. Target.Ther.* **9** 175
[26] Turajlic S, Sottoriva A, Graham T and Swanton C 2019 Resolving genetic heterogeneity in cancer *Nat. Rev. Genet.* **20** 404–16
[27] Gilbert A, Bonny M and Arisen H 2024 *Research Square* 10.21203/rs.3.rs-5553130/v1 03 December 2024 A systematic review of the imaging modalities used for image acquisition https://doi.org/10.21203/rs.3.rs-5553130/v1
[28] Hussain T and Nguyen Q T 2014 Molecular imaging for cancer diagnosis and surgery *Adv. Drug Deliv. Rev.* **66** 90–100
[29] Singh A, Handa V, Kaur H, Likhitkar S, Singh R S and Medhi B 2023 Strategies of early diagnosis of cancers *Handbook of Oncobiology: From Basic to Clinical Sciences* (Berlin: Springer) pp 1–20

[30] Pulumati A, Pulumati A, Dwarakanath B S, Verma A and Papineni R V 2023 Technological advancements in cancer diagnostics: improvements and limitations *Cancer Rep.* **6** e1764

[31] Cescon D W, Bratman S V, Chan S M and Siu L L 2020 Circulating tumor DNA and liquid biopsy in oncology *Nat. Cancer* **1** 276–90

[32] 2015 *Improving diagnosis in health care* ed E P Balogh, B T Miller and J R Ball (Washington (DC): National Academies Press (US))

[33] Weller D, Vedsted P, Rubin G, Walter F, Emery J, Scott S, Campbell C, Andersen R S, Hamilton W and Olesen F 2012 The Aarhus statement: improving design and reporting of studies on early cancer diagnosis *Br. J. Cancer* **106** 1262–7

[34] Kroenke K 2014 A practical and evidence-based approach to common symptoms: a narrative review *Ann. Int. Med.* **161** 579–86

[35] Sawicki T, Ruszkowska M, Danielewicz A, Niedźwiedzka E, Arłukowicz T and Przybyłowicz K E 2021 A review of colorectal cancer in terms of epidemiology, risk factors, development, symptoms and diagnosis *Cancers* **13** 2025

[36] Singh H, Sethi S, Raber M and Petersen L A 2007 Errors in cancer diagnosis: current understanding and future directions *J. Clin. Oncol.* **25** 5009–18

[37] Al-Worafi Y M, Ming L C and Alseragi W M 2024 Patient Care-Related Issues in the Developing Countries: Patient Education and Counseling *Handbook of Medical and Health Sciences in Developing Countries* ed Y M Al-Worafi (Cham: Springer)

[38] Meric-Bernstam F and Mills G B 2012 Overcoming implementation challenges of personalized cancer therapy *Nat. Rev. Clin. Oncol.* **9** 542–8

[39] Vallabani N V, Singh S and Karakoti A S 2019 Magnetic nanoparticles: current trends and future aspects in diagnostics and nanomedicine *Curr. Drug Metab.* **20** 457–72

[40] Araújo E, Carneiro S, Neto D, Freire T, Costa V, Freire R, Fechine L, Clemente C, Denardin J and Dos Santos J 2024 Advances in surface design and biomedical applications of magnetic nanoparticles *Adv. Colloid Interface Sci.* **328** 103166

[41] Rezaei B, Yari P, Sanders S M, Wang H, Chugh V K, Liang S, Mostufa S, Xu K, Wang J P and Gómez-Pastora J 2024 Magnetic nanoparticles: a review on synthesis, characterization, functionalization, and biomedical applications *Small* **20** 2304848

[42] Shakeri-Zadeh A and Bulte J W 2024 Imaging-guided precision hyperthermia with magnetic nanoparticles *Nat. Rev. Bioeng.* **3** 245–60

[43] Ko M J, Min S, Hong H, Yoo W, Joo J, Zhang Y S, Kang H and Kim D-H 2024 Magnetic nanoparticles for ferroptosis cancer therapy with diagnostic imaging *Bioact. Mater.* **32** 66–97

[44] Zhuo Y, Zhao Y-G and Zhang Y 2024 Enhancing drug solubility, bioavailability, and targeted therapeutic applications through magnetic nanoparticles *Molecules* **29** 4854

[45] Mhlanga N, Mphuthi N, Van der Walt H, Nyembe S, Mokhena T and Sikhwivhilu L 2024 Nanostructures and nanoparticles as medical diagnostic imaging contrast agents: a review *Mater. Today Chem.* **40** 102233

[46] Tryphena K P, Kulkarni A, Rajan S, Jain R, Pasupuleti V and Khatri D K 2025 Functionalized magnetic nanoparticles for photoacoustics and ultrasound imaging *Functionalized Magnetic Nanoparticles for Theranostic Applications* (Austin, TX: Scrivener Publishing LLC) pp 503–32

[47] Rezaei B, Tay Z, Mostufa S, Manzari O N, Azizi E, Ciannella S, Li C, Zeng M, Gomez-Pastora J and Wu K 2024 Magnetic nanoparticles for magnetic particle imaging (MPI): design and applications *Nanoscale* **16** 11802–24

[48] Butt A and Bach H 2024 Advancements in nanotechnology for diagnostics: a literature review, part II: advanced techniques in nuclear and optical imaging *Nanomedicine* **20** 183–206
[49] Luo G-F and Zhang X-Z 2024 Magnetic nanoparticles for use in bioimaging *Biomater. Sci.* **12** 6224–36
[50] Shin T-H, Choi Y, Kim S and Cheon J 2015 Recent advances in magnetic nanoparticle-based multimodal imaging *Chem. Soc. Rev.* **44** 4501–16
[51] Abhisheka B, Biswas S K, Purkayastha B, Das D and Escargueil A 2024 Recent trend in medical imaging modalities and their applications in disease diagnosis: a review *Multimed. Tools Appl.* **83** 43035–70
[52] Li K-R, Wu A-G, Tang Y, He X-P, Yu C-L, Wu J-M, Hu G-Q and Yu L 2022 The key role of magnetic resonance imaging in the detection of neurodegenerative diseases-associated biomarkers: a review *Mol. Neurobiol.* **59** 5935–54
[53] Dhabalia R, Kashikar S V, Parihar P S and Mishra G V 2024 Unveiling the intricacies: a comprehensive review of magnetic resonance imaging (MRI) assessment of T2-weighted hyperintensities in the neuroimaging landscape *Cureus* **16** e54808
[54] Summers P, Saia G, Colombo A, Pricolo P, Zugni F, Alessi S, Marvaso G, Jereczek-Fossa B A, Bellomi M and Petralia G 2021 Whole-body magnetic resonance imaging: technique, guidelines and key applications *Ecancermedicalscience* **15** 1164
[55] Hussain S, Mubeen I, Ullah N, Shah S S U D, Khan B A, Zahoor M, Ullah R, Khan F A and Sultan M A 2022 Modern diagnostic imaging technique applications and risk factors in the medical field: a review *BioMed Res. Int.* **2022** 5164970
[56] Sun C, Lee J S and Zhang M 2008 Magnetic nanoparticles in MR imaging and drug delivery *Adv. Drug Deliv. Rev.* **60** 1252–65
[57] Geraldes C F 2024 Rational design of magnetic nanoparticles as T1–T2 dual-mode MRI contrast agents *Molecules* **29** 1352
[58] Yallapu M M, Othman S F, Curtis E T, Gupta B K, Jaggi M and Chauhan S C 2011 Multi-functional magnetic nanoparticles for magnetic resonance imaging and cancer therapy *Biomaterials* **32** 1890–905
[59] Govindan B, Sabri M A, Hai A, Banat F and Haija M A 2023 A review of advanced multifunctional magnetic nanostructures for cancer diagnosis and therapy integrated into an artificial intelligence approach *Pharmaceutics* **15** 868
[60] Farinha P, Coelho J M, Reis C P and Gaspar M M 2021 A comprehensive updated review on magnetic nanoparticles in diagnostics *Nanomaterials* **11** 3432
[61] Antwi-Baah R, Wang Y, Chen X and Yu K 2022 Metal-based nanoparticle magnetic resonance imaging contrast agents: classifications, issues, and countermeasures toward their clinical translation *Adv. Mater. Interfaces* **9** 2101710
[62] Zhang W, Liu L, Chen H, Hu K, Delahunty I, Gao S and Xie J 2018 Surface impact on nanoparticle-based magnetic resonance imaging contrast agents *Theranostics* **8** 2521
[63] Cardoso V F, Francesko A, Ribeiro C, Bañobre-López M, Martins P and Lanceros-Mendez S 2018 Advances in magnetic nanoparticles for biomedical applications *Adv. Healthcare Mater.* **7** 1700845
[64] Barua S and Mitragotri S 2014 Challenges associated with penetration of nanoparticles across cell and tissue barriers: a review of current status and future prospects *Nano Today* **9** 223–43

[65] Ryapolov P, Vasilyeva A, Kalyuzhnaya D, Churaev A, Sokolov E and Shel'deshova E 2024 Magnetic fluids: the interaction between the microstructure, macroscopic properties, and dynamics under different combinations of external influences *Nanomaterials* **14** 222
[66] Truong T T, Mondal S, Doan V H M, Tak S, Choi J, Oh H, Nguyen T D, Misra M, Lee B and Oh J 2024 Precision-engineered metal and metal-oxide nanoparticles for biomedical imaging and healthcare applications *Adv. Colloid Interface Sci.* **332** 103263
[67] Kang T, Li F, Baik S, Shao W, Ling D and Hyeon T 2017 Surface design of magnetic nanoparticles for stimuli-responsive cancer imaging and therapy *Biomaterials* **136** 98–114
[68] Yin C, Hu P, Qin L, Wang Z and Zhao H 2024 The current status and future directions on nanoparticles for tumor molecular imaging *Int. J. Nanomed.* **19** 9549–74
[69] Abbas Q, Zia-ur-Rehman M, Ullah H, Munir M A M, Ali M U, Ali A, Pikon K and Yousaf B 2024 Recent advances in the detection and quantification of manufactured nanoparticles (MNPs) in complex environmental and biological matrices *J. Clean. Prod.* **471** 143454
[70] Fang J, Nakamura H and Maeda H 2011 The EPR effect: unique features of tumor blood vessels for drug delivery, factors involved, and limitations and augmentation of the effect *Adv. Drug Deliv. Rev.* **63** 136–51
[71] Popov A L, Savintseva I V, Kozlova T O, Ivanova O S, Zhukov I V, Baranchikov A E, Yurkovskaya A V, Savelov A A, Ermakov A M and Popova N R 2023 Heavily Gd-doped non-toxic cerium oxide nanoparticles for MRI labelling of stem cells *Molecules* **28** 1165
[72] Iyer A K, He J and Amiji M M 2012 Image-guided nanosystems for targeted delivery in cancer therapy *Curr. Med. Chem.* **19** 3230–40
[73] Taboada E, Rodríguez E, Roig A, Oró J, Roch A and Muller R N 2007 Relaxometric and magnetic characterization of ultrasmall iron oxide nanoparticles with high magnetization. Evaluation as potential T1 magnetic resonance imaging contrast agents for molecular imaging *Langmuir* **23** 4583–8
[74] Yue H, Zhao D, Tegafaw T, Ahmad M Y, Saidi A K A A, Liu Y, Cha H, Yang B W, Chae K S, Nam S-W *et al* 2024 Core–shell Fe_3O_4@C nanoparticles as highly effective T2 magnetic resonance imaging contrast agents: *in vitro* and *in vivo* studies *Nanomaterials* **14** 177
[75] Al-Thani A N, Jan A G, Abbas M, Geetha M and Sadasivuni K K 2024 Nanoparticles in cancer theragnostic and drug delivery: a comprehensive review *Life Sci.* **352** 122899
[76] Materón E M, Miyazaki C M, Carr O, Joshi N, Picciani P H S, Dalmaschio C J, Davis F and Shimizu F M 2021 Magnetic nanoparticles in biomedical applications: a review *Appl. Surf. Sci. Adv.* **6** 100163
[77] Yu J, Ju Y, Chen F, Che S, Zhao L, Sheng F and Hou Y 2018 Chemical synthesis and biomedical applications of iron oxide nanoparticles *Nanobiomaterials: Classification, Fabrication and Biomedical Applications* (New York: Wiley) pp 329–58
[78] Maier A, Jia Q, Shukla K, Dugulan A I, Hagedoorn P-L, van Oossanen R, van Rhoon G, Denkova A G and Djanashvili K 2024 Enhancing magnetic hyperthermia efficiency in Pd/Fe-oxide hybrid nanoparticles through Mn-doping *ACS Appl. Nano Mater.* **7** 27465–75
[79] Sikma R E, Reyes R A, Richards D, Kotula P G, Meyerson M L, Schafer D P, Romàn-Kustas J K, Percival S J and Sava Gallis D F 2024 Monodisperse Cu nanoparticles supported on a versatile metal–organic framework for electrocatalytic reduction of CO_2 *ACS Appl. Nano Mater.* **7** 26629–35

[80] Patel S, McKelvey K and Liu L 2024 Metal–organic frameworks for electrocatalytic CO_2 reduction: developments and prospects *Chem. Mater.* **36** 10054–87

[81] Glasby L T, Cordiner J L, Cole J C and Moghadam P Z 2024 Topological characterization of metal–organic frameworks: a perspective *Chem. Mater.* **36** 9013–30

[82] Khosla A, Wani I A and Lone M N 2025 Biomedical applications of iron-oxide-based magnetic nanoparticles *Metallic, Magnetic, and Carbon-Based Nanomaterials: Synthesis and Biomedical Applications* (New York: Wiley) pp 171–235

[83] Hao R, Xing R, Xu Z, Hou Y, Gao S and Sun S 2010 Synthesis, functionalization, and biomedical applications of multifunctional magnetic nanoparticles *Adv. Mater.* **22** 2729–42

[84] Yang H Y, Li Y and Lee D S 2021 Functionalization of magnetic nanoparticles with organic ligands toward biomedical applications *Adv. NanoBiomed Res.* **1** 2000043

[85] Unterweger H, Janko C, Folk T, Cicha I, Kovács N, Gyebnár G, Horváth I, Máthé D, Zheng K H and Coolen B F 2023 Comparative *in vitro* and *in vivo* evaluation of different iron oxide-based contrast agents to promote clinical translation in compliance with patient safety *Int. J. Nanomed.* 2071–86

[86] Chan M-H, Hsieh M-R, Liu R-S, Wei D-H and Hsiao M 2020 Magnetically guided theranostics: optimizing magnetic resonance imaging with sandwich-like kaolinite-based iron/platinum nanoparticles for magnetic fluid hyperthermia and chemotherapy *Chem. Mater.* **32** 697–708

[87] Xiao Y, Lin Z T, Chen Y, Wang H, Deng Y L, Le D E, Bin J, Li M, Liao Y and Liu Y 2015 High molecular weight chitosan derivative polymeric micelles encapsulating superparamagnetic iron oxide for tumor-targeted magnetic resonance imaging *Int. J. Nanomed.* **10** 1155–72

[88] Xie H, Zhu Y, Jiang W, Zhou Q, Yang H, Gu N, Zhang Y, Xu H, Xu H and Yang X 2011 Lactoferrin-conjugated superparamagnetic iron oxide nanoparticles as a specific MRI contrast agent for detection of brain glioma *in vivo Biomaterials* **32** 495–502

[89] Gonzalez-Rodriguez R, Campbell E and Naumov A 2019 Multifunctional graphene oxide/iron oxide nanoparticles for magnetic targeted drug delivery dual magnetic resonance/fluorescence imaging and cancer sensing *PLoS One* **14** e0217072

[90] Zhang Y, Zhang L, Song X, Gu X, Sun H, Fu C and Meng F 2015 Synthesis of superparamagnetic iron oxide nanoparticles modified with MPEG-PEI via photochemistry as New MRI contrast agent *J. Nanomater.* **2015** 417389

[91] Ding X, Liu J, Li J, Wang F, Wang Y, Song S and Zhang H 2016 Polydopamine coated manganese oxide nanoparticles with ultrahigh relaxivity as nanotheranostic agents for magnetic resonance imaging guided synergetic chemo-/photothermal therapy *Chem. Sci.* **7** 6695–700

[92] Geraldes C F G C 2024 Manganese oxide nanoparticles for MRI-based multimodal imaging and theranostics *Molecules* **29** 5591

[93] Bu L, Shen B and Cheng Z 2014 Fluorescent imaging of cancerous tissues for targeted surgery *Adv. Drug Deliv. Rev.* **76** 21–38

[94] Wang K, Liu C, Zhu H, Zhang Y, Su M, Wang X, Liu M, Rong X and Zhu B 2023 Recent advances in small-molecule fluorescent probes for diagnosis of cancer cells/tissues *Coord. Chem. Rev.* **477** 214946

[95] Seah D, Cheng Z and Vendrell M 2023 Fluorescent probes for imaging in humans: where are we now? *ACS Nano* **17** 19478–90

[96] Luo H and Gao S 2023 Recent advances in fluorescence imaging-guided photothermal therapy and photodynamic therapy for cancer: from near-infrared-I to near-infrared-II *J. Control. Release* **362** 425–45

[97] Kravchenko Y, Sikora K, Wireko A A and Lyndin M 2024 Fluorescence visualization for cancer detection: experience and perspectives *Heliyon* **10** e24390

[98] Woo Y, Chaurasiya S, O'Leary M, Han E and Fong Y 2021 Fluorescent imaging for cancer therapy and cancer gene therapy *Mol. Ther.—Oncol.* **23** 231–8

[99] Kanno H, Hiramatsu K, Mikami H, Nakayashiki A, Yamashita S, Nagai A, Okabe K, Li F, Yin F, Tominaga K *et al* 2024 High-throughput fluorescence lifetime imaging flow cytometry *Nat. Commun.* **15** 7376

[100] Malik M M U D, Alqahtani M M, Hadadi I, Kanbayti I, Alawaji Z and Aloufi B A 2024 Molecular imaging biomarkers for early cancer detection: a systematic review of emerging technologies and clinical applications *Diagnostics* **14** 2459

[101] Passaro A, Al Bakir M, Hamilton E G, Diehn M, André F, Roy-Chowdhuri S, Mountzios G, Wistuba I I, Swanton C and Peters S 2024 Cancer biomarkers: emerging trends and clinical implications for personalized treatment *Cell* **187** 1617–35

[102] Sun M, Sun B, Liu Y, Shen Q-D and Jiang S 2016 Dual-color fluorescence imaging of magnetic nanoparticles in live cancer cells using conjugated polymer probes *Sci. Rep.* **6** 22368

[103] Tang J L Y, Moonshi S S, Wu Y, Cowin G, Vazquez- Prada K X, Tran H D N, Bulmer A C and Ta H T 2025 A methotrexate labelled dual metal oxide nanocomposite for long-lasting anti-cancer theranostics *Mater. Today Bio* **30** 101377

[104] Ahmed M, Ibrahim M, Elbashir F E M, Bagdadi N and Awad F 2024 Iron oxide nanoparticles functionalized with macrocycle antagonists for CXCR4 receptor targeting in cancer cells *J. Anal. Oncol.* **13** 36–42

[105] Fu A, Wilson R J, Smith B R, Mullenix J, Earhart C, Akin D, Guccione S, Wang S X and Gambhir S S 2012 Fluorescent magnetic nanoparticles for magnetically enhanced cancer imaging and targeting in living subjects *ACS Nano* **6** 6862–9

[106] Divband B, Gharehaghaji N and Hassani S 2022 Fe_3O_4/graphene-based nanotheranostics for bimodal magnetic resonance/fluorescence imaging and cancer therapy *J. Inorg. Organomet. Polym. Mater.* **32** 4443–60

[107] Zou X, Lin R, Fu Y, Gong G, Zhou X, Wang S, Zhu S and Wang Z 2024 Advanced optical imaging based on metasurfaces *Adv. Opt. Mater.* **12** 2203149

[108] Dey S, Dolci M and Zijlstra P 2023 Single-molecule optical biosensing: recent advances and future challenges *ACS Phys. Chem. Au* **3** 143–56

[109] Rasheed S, Kanwal T, Ahmad N, Fatima B, Najam-ul-Haq M and Hussain D 2024 Advances and challenges in portable optical biosensors for onsite detection and point-of-care diagnostics *TrAC, Trends Anal. Chem.* **173** 117640

[110] Xiang M, Liu F, Liu J, Dong X, Liu Q and Shao X 2024 Computational optical imaging: challenges, opportunities, new trends, and emerging applications *Front. Imag.* **3** 1336829

[111] Yan X, Song X and Wang Z 2017 Construction of specific magnetic resonance imaging/optical dual-modality molecular probe used for imaging angiogenesis of gastric cancer *Artif. Cells, Nanomed. Biotechnol.* **45** 399–403

[112] Luengo Morato Y, Ovejero Paredes K, Lozano Chamizo L, Marciello M and Filice M 2021 Recent advances in multimodal molecular imaging of cancer mediated by hybrid magnetic nanoparticles *Polymers (Basel)* **13** 2989

[113] Zhang L, Wang Y, Peng Z, Weng Y, Fang Z, Xiao F, Zhang C, Fan Z, Huang K, Zhu Y *et al* 2022 The progress of multimodal imaging combination and subregion based radiomics research of cancers *Int. J. Biol. Sci.* **18** 3458–69
[114] Song L, Liu S and Liu X 2023 Chapter 4—Learning from multiple modalities of imaging data for cancer diagnosis *Computational Intelligence in Cancer Diagnosis* ed J Nayak, D Pelusi, B Naik, M Mishra, K Muhammad and D Al-Dabass (New York: Academic) pp 67–87
[115] Wang S, Liu M, Li Y, Zhang X, Sun M, Wang Z, Li R, Li Q, Li Q, He Y *et al* 2025 Recent advances in data-driven fusion of multimodal imaging and genomics for precision medicine *Inform. Fusion* **115** 102738
[116] Wang L, Wan Q, Zhang R, Situ B, Ni K, Gao J, Feng X, Zhang P, Wang Z, Qin A *et al* 2021 Synergistic enhancement of fluorescence and magnetic resonance signals assisted by albumin aggregate for dual-modal imaging *ACS Nano* **15** 9924–34
[117] Kuang S, Wan Y, Dai Y, Mo C, Fei Y, Shi J, Han C and Huang T 2025 Multifunctional molecular theranostic agent for fluorescence-magnetic resonance dual-modal imaging and photodynamic-chemodynamic synergistic therapy *Sens. Actuators* B **426** 137035
[118] Mukherjee S, Liang L and Veiseh O 2020 Recent advancements of magnetic nanomaterials in cancer therapy *Pharmaceutics* **12** 147
[119] Graziotto M E, Kidman C J, Adair L D, James S A, Harris H H and New E J 2023 Towards multimodal cellular imaging: optical and X-ray fluorescence *Chem. Soc. Rev.* **52** 8295–318
[120] Thomas R, Park I-K and Jeong Y Y 2013 Magnetic iron oxide nanoparticles for multimodal imaging and therapy of cancer *Int. J. Mol. Sci.* **14** 15910–30
[121] Sobhanan J, Anas A and Biju V 2023 Nanomaterials for fluorescence and multimodal bioimaging *Chem. Rec.* **23** e202200253
[122] Pan Q, Ye S, Yang D, Qiu J and Dong G 2017 Multifunctional magnetic-fluorescent Ni-doped ZnAl2O4 nanoparticles with second biological NIR window fluorescence *Mater. Res. Bull.* **93** 310–7
[123] Hu H, Sheng Y, Ye M, Qian Y, Tang J and Shen Y 2016 A porphyrin-based magnetic and fluorescent dual-modal nanoprobe for tumor imaging *Polymer* **88** 94–101
[124] Zhang L, Tong S, Zhang Q and Bao G 2020 Lipid-encapsulated Fe_3O_4 nanoparticles for multimodal magnetic resonance/fluorescence imaging *ACS Appl. Nano Mater.* **3** 6785–97
[125] Zhang L, Tong S, Zhang Q and Bao G 2020 Lipid-Encapsulated Fe_3O_4 Nanoparticles for Multimodal Magnetic Resonance/Fluorescence Imaging *Appl. Nano Mater.* **3** 6785–97
[126] Bao J, Guo S, Zu X, Zhuang Y, Fan D, Zhang Y, Shi Y, Pang X, Ji Z and Cheng J 2022 Magnetic vortex nanoring coated with gadolinium oxide for highly enhanced T1-T2 dual-modality magnetic resonance imaging-guided magnetic hyperthermia cancer ablation *Biomed. Pharmacother.* **150** 112926
[127] Xue F, Zhu S, Tian Q, Qin R, Wang Z, Huang G and Yang S 2023 Macrophage-mediated delivery of magnetic nanoparticles for enhanced magnetic resonance imaging and magneto-thermal therapy of solid tumors *J. Colloid Interface Sci.* **629** 554–62
[128] Xue S, Wang Y, Wang M, Zhang L, Du X, Gu H and Zhang C 2014 Iodinated oil-loaded, fluorescent mesoporous silica-coated iron oxide nanoparticles for magnetic resonance imaging/computed tomography/fluorescence trimodal imaging *Int. J. Nanomed.* **9** 2527–38
[129] Wu B, Wan B, Lu S-T, Deng K, Li X-Q, Wu B-L, Li Y-S, Liao R-F, Huang S-W and Xu H-B 2017 Near-infrared light-triggered theranostics for tumor-specific enhanced multimodal imaging and photothermal therapy *Int. J. Nanomed.* **12** 4467–78

[130] Deng X, Dai Y, Liu J, Zhou Y, Ma P A, Cheng Z, Chen Y, Deng K, Li X, Hou Z *et al* 2015 Multifunctional hollow $CaF_2:Yb^{3+}/Er^{3+}/Mn^{2+}$-poly(2-aminoethyl methacrylate) microspheres for Pt(IV) pro-drug delivery and tri-modal imaging *Biomaterials* **50** 154–63

[131] Yang G, Gong H, Liu T, Sun X, Cheng L and Liu Z 2015 Two-dimensional magnetic $WS_2@Fe_3O_4$ nanocomposite with mesoporous silica coating for drug delivery and imaging-guided therapy of cancer *Biomaterials* **60** 62–71

[132] Dong W, Li Y, Niu D, Ma Z, Liu X, Gu J, Zhao W, Zheng Y and Shi J 2013 A simple route to prepare monodisperse Au NP-decorated, dye-doped, superparamagnetic nanocomposites for optical, MR, and CT trimodal imaging *Small* **9** 2500–8

[133] Han L, Xia J-M, Hai X, Shu Y, Chen X-W and Wang J-H 2017 Protein-stabilized gadolinium oxide-gold nanoclusters hybrid for multimodal imaging and drug delivery *ACS Appl. Mater. Interfaces* **9** 6941–9

[134] Li H, Parigi G, Luchinat C and Meade T J 2019 Bimodal fluorescence-magnetic resonance contrast agent for apoptosis imaging *J. Am. Chem. Soc.* **141** 6224–33

[135] Zain M, Yasmeen H, Yadav S S, Amir S, Bilal M, Shahid A and Khurshid M 2022 Chapter 10—Applications of nanotechnology in biological systems and medicine *Nanotechnology for Hematology, Blood Transfusion, and Artificial Blood* ed A Denizli, T A Nguyen, M Rajan, M F Alam and K Rahman (Amsterdam: Elsevier) pp 215–35

IOP Publishing

Magnetic Nanomaterials

Innovation for cancer theranostics

Sudip Mukherjee, Vijay Sagar Madamsetty, Lipi Pradhan, Anjali Upadhyay and Devyani Yenurkar

Chapter 5

MNPs in clinical trials

Advancements in nanotechnology have successfully translated oncological research into clinical practice, improving cancer diagnosis and management. Several nanoscale products have received US Food and Drug Administration (FDA) approval and are currently available. Today, scientists are exploring the theranostic potential of magnetic nanoparticles (MNPs) in cancer nanomedicine by integrating the diagnostic and therapeutic potentials of MNPs. Various MNPs are currently used in clinical practice as contrast-enhancing agents in imaging techniques such as magnetic resonance imaging (MRI). This chapter provides a comprehensive overview of recent clinical trials involving various MNPs in cancer theranostics, highlighting both clinical trials and approved applications.

The incidence and mortality rates of cancer are proliferating, making it a significant health concern across the world and imposing emotional and economic burdens on patients and their loved ones [1–4]. The International Agency for Research on Cancer (IARC) published the GLOBOCAN 2020 database, which estimated that 19.3 million new cases of cancer were reported globally in 2020, leading to almost 10 million deaths. According to projections, the number of cancer cases worldwide is expected to rise by 47% from 2020 to about 28.4 million cases by 2040 [5, 6]. The urgent need for improved cancer prevention, early detection, and treatment strategies is highlighted by this concerning trend. For a long time, traditional cancer therapies have been used; however, they frequently come with substantial drawbacks and adverse consequences [7]. This has led to considerable study aimed at creating novel therapeutic approaches.

Nanotechnology-based techniques, collectively known as cancer nanomedicine, have emerged due to the inherent limitations of conventional treatments [8]. Advancements in nanotechnology have successfully translated oncological research into clinical practice, improving cancer diagnosis and management. Several nanoscale products have received FDA approval and are currently available on the market [9]. Despite massive progress in cancer management and research, current

doi:10.1088/978-0-7503-6335-8ch5

© IOP Publishing Ltd 2025. All rights, including for text and data mining (TDM), artificial intelligence (AI) training, and similar technologies, are reserved.

treatment approaches can only provide patients with limited health and survival benefits.

Scientists are currently exploring the theranostic potential of MNPs in cancer nanomedicine by integrating the diagnostic and therapeutic potentials of MNPs. Numerous physicochemical properties of MNPs make them suitable for a variety of biomedical applications, including targeted drug delivery, imaging, and hyperthermic therapies, highlighting their potential as a transformative tool in cancer nanomedicine [10–14]. Early clinical results have demonstrated that MNPs can outperform conventional therapies by offering improved therapeutic efficacy and reduced side effects, as they target the affected area without damaging nearby tissues [15, 16]. The application of MNPs as a treatment option for cancer was first proposed in 1970 to target tumors [17]. After that, they were studied for various applications in cancer theranostics. Various MNPs are currently used in clinical practice as contrast-enhancing agents in imaging techniques such as MRI [18–20]. Due to their distinctive characteristics, MNPs can have dual roles in cancer treatment: they can serve as drug delivery systems that preferentially deliver drugs to cancerous lesions while also functioning as imaging probes to identify and diagnose those lesions. These two capabilities are currently being combined to create MNP-based nanotheranostics with imaging and therapeutic capabilities that will support the growth of personalized medicine and allow for real-time tracking of the body's response to treatment [21]. The primary objectives of ongoing clinical trials involving MNPs are diagnostic applications and the creation of hyperthermia to eliminate tumors. Early clinical trials are in progress for multiple types of MNPs, and some compositions have received clinical approval for use in therapeutic and medical imaging applications. Among these, Gastromark® and Lumiren® are employed for bowel imaging, whereas Endorem® and Feridex I.V.® are approved for imaging of the spleen and liver [15].

MNPs have attracted significant attention in cancer theranostics as targeted drug delivery systems with enhanced biocompatibility, reduced systemic toxicity, and increased drug accumulation at the desired location. Furthermore, the application of a magnetic field can lead to hyperthermia in MNPs, which either directly causes cancer cell death or triggers the release of drugs from thermoresponsive magnetic carriers [22, 23]. Recent experimental investigations have extensively employed MNPs in cancer therapy, developing various magnetic formulations. These formulations have shown promising therapeutic effects across a range of cancer types, highlighting the potential of MNPs in advancing personalized and effective cancer treatments. This chapter offers a complete overview of recent clinical trials of various MNPs in cancer theranostics, highlighting both clinical trials and approved applications. Additionally, we explore multiple patents recently published on the use of MNPs in cancer theranostics. Further sections of this chapter deal with the clinical outcomes of these trials, assessing their current applicability and success rates. This analysis aims to highlight the practical effectiveness of MNPs in real-life scenarios, demonstrating the potential of MNPs to revolutionize cancer theranostics. The recently published clinical trials of MNPs are summarized in table 5.1.

Table 5.1. Clinical trials of MNPs for cancer theranostics.

Sl. No.	Company/ institution	Intervention	Investigated application	Phase	Recruitment status	Study completion date	NCT (National Clinical Trial) number	References
1.	University College London Hospitals	MNP injection	MNP thermoablation for the management of prostate cancer	Early phase 1	Completed	January 2015	NCT02033447	[24]
2.	University of Zurich	MNP	Detection of blood tumor cells using MNPs		Completed	30 December 2022	NCT04290923	[25–27]
3.	Västra Götaland Region	MagTrace and Magseed	Identification of axillary lymph node before neoadjuvant chemotherapy in breast cancer patients		Completed	28 November 2023	NCT05625698	[28–31]
4.	Uppsala University	Sentinel lymph node detection or targeted axillary dissection by the magnetic technique super paramagnetic iron oxide (SPIO)	Feasibility of SLND by SPIO in early breast cancer patients		Active, not recruiting	30 October 2027 (estimated)	NCT05985551	[32, 33]

(*Continued*)

Table 5.1. (*Continued*)

Sl. No.	Company/ institution	Intervention	Investigated application	Phase	Recruitment status	Study completion date	NCT (National Clinical Trial) number	References
5.	Sahlgrenska University Hospital	Superparamagnetic iron oxide (MagTrace)	Sentinel node localization with low dose SPIO-enhanced MRI and magnetic probe in breast cancer patients	Phase 1 Phase 2	Active, not recruiting	30 April 2024 (estimated)	NCT05359783	[34–37]
6.	Uppsala University	Diagnostic tests using super paramagnetic iron oxide nanoparticles (SPIONs)	SPIONs for the detection of breast cancer	Phase 3	Recruiting	30 December 2027 (estimated)	NCT04722692	[33]
7.	Allegheny Singer Research Institute	Ferumoxytol injection	Treatment of hepatic cancers using radiotherapy with SPIONs in magnetic-resonance-guided linear accelerator (MR-linac)		Active, not recruiting	31 December 2024 (estimated)	NCT04682847	

8.	M.D. Anderson Cancer Center	Ferumoxytol	MNPs as contrast agent in MRI for imaging head and neck tumors	Early phase 1	Terminated		NCT01895829	[38]
9.	University of New Mexico	Magnetic needle (MagProbe)	Magnetic needle containing iron oxide nanoparticles (IONPs) for the detection of leukemia		Withdrawn		NCT01411904	[39]
10.	Dana-Farber Cancer Institute	AGuIX, a gadolinium-based nanoparticle	Treatment of lung and pancreatic tumor using gadolinium-based nanoparticles with magnetic-resonance-guided stereotactic body radiotherapy (MR-guided SBRT)	Phase 1 Phase 2	Recruiting	10 September 2027	NCT04789486	[40]
11.	Saving Patients' Lives Medical B.V.	Ferrotran® (Ferumoxtran-10)	Prostate cancer diagnosis by ferumoxtran-10-enhanced MRI	Phase 3	Active, not recruiting	January 2025 (estimated)	NCT04261777	[41–44]

(*Continued*)

Table 5.1. (*Continued*)

Sl. No.	Company/ institution	Intervention	Investigated application	Phase	Recruitment status	Study completion date	NCT (National Clinical Trial) number	References
12.	University Hospital, Grenoble	AGuIX (nanosized gadolinium particles)	AGuIX for radio sensitization of multiple brain metastases	Phase 1	Completed	February 2019	NCT02820454	[45]
13.	Centre Francois Baclesse	AGuIX® nanoparticles.	Hypofractionated proton therapy with MNPs for reirradiation of pancreatic tumor relapse	Phase 2	Not yet recruiting	September 2027 (estimated)	NCT04784221	
14.	University Hospital, Grenoble	AGuIX® (gadolinium-chelated polysiloxane-based nanoparticles/ NANORAD2)	Radiotherapy using AGuIX® for treatment of multiple brain tumors	Phase 2	Active, not recruiting	26 March 2025 (estimated)	NCT03818386	[46–48]
15.	Centre Jean Perrin	Polysiloxane Gd-chelate-based nanoparticles (AGuIX)	Treatment of newly diagnosed glioblastoma using concomitant temozolomide, AGuIX, and radiotherapy	Phase 1/2	Active, not recruiting	March 2027 (estimated)	NCT04881032	[49]

16.	Dana-Farber Cancer Institute	AGuIX (gadolinium-based nanoparticles)	Brain metastases treated with SBRT and AGuIX	Phase 2	Recruiting	February 2026 (estimated)	NCT04899908	
17.	Zhejiang University	neoadjuvant chemotherapy + SPIONs/spinning magnetic field (SMF)	Neoadjuvant chemotherapy with/without SPIONs/SMF for patients with osteosarcoma	Phase I	Unknown status	31 August 2023 (estimated)	NCT04316091	[50]
18.	Poznan University of Medical Sciences	NanoTherm therapy	MNPs as adjuvant therapy for cyclic hyperthermia in patients with glioblastoma multiforme (GBM)		Recruiting	01 September 2027 (estimated)	NCT06271421	[51–55]
19.	Nanobiotix	NBTXR3 activated by intensity-modulated radiation therapy (IMRT)	Activation of NBTXR3 by radiation therapy in patients suffering from squamous cell carcinoma of the oropharynx or oral cavity	Phase I	Unknown status	February 2023 (estimated)	NCT01946867	[56]

(*Continued*)

Table 5.1. (*Continued*)

Sl. No.	Company/ institution	Intervention	Investigated application	Phase	Recruitment status	Study completion date	NCT (National Clinical Trial) number	References
20.	Gustave Roussy, Cancer Campus, Grand Paris	Polysiloxane Gd-chelate-based nanoparticles (AGuIX)	AGuIX with chemoradiation and brachytherapy in locally advanced cervical cancer	Phase 1	Unknown status	May 2024 (estimated)	NCT03308604	[57]
21.	Nanobiotix	NBTXR3	Liver cancer treatment using NBTXR3 activated by SBRT	Phase 1 Phase 2	Terminated	06 May 2020	NCT02721056	
22.	Nanobiotix	NBTXR3	NBTXR3 activated by radiotherapy for patients with advanced cancers	Phase 1	Recruiting	30 May 2028 (estimated)	NCT03589339	[58]
23.	Nanobiotix	NBTXR3	Patients with soft tissue tumors of the extremities and trunk walls treated with NBTXR3 as an intratumoral	Phase 2 Phase 3	Completed	20 September 2020	NCT02379845	[59]

			injection and radiation therapy					
24.	M.D. Anderson Cancer Center	Hafnium-oxide-containing nanoparticles, NBTXR3	Radiation therapy-activated NBTXR3 for the management of pancreatic cancer	Phase 1	Recruiting	31 December 2026 (estimated)	NCT04484909	[60]
25.	M.D. Anderson Cancer Center	Hafnium-oxide-containing nanoparticles, NBTXR3	Radiation therapy combined with concurrent chemotherapy to activate NBTXR3 in esophageal adeno carcinoma	Phase 1	Recruiting	31 October 2025 (estimated)	NCT04615013	
26.	M.D. Anderson Cancer Center	Hafnium-oxide-containing nanoparticles, NBTXR3	Treatment of lung cancer using NBTXR3 and radiation therapy	Phase 1	Recruiting	31 March 2026 (estimated)	NCT04505267	

5.1 Clinical trials of MNPs for imaging and diagnosis of cancer

Imaging-based diagnosis plays a vital role in the management of cancer. It helps to identify the severity of the cancer, plan suitable therapy, and observe the patient's response to treatment. There are various imaging tests available on the market, which include ultrasound (US), positron emission tomography (PET), MRI, single-photon emission computed tomography (SPECT), photoacoustic (PA) imaging, computed tomography (CT), optical fluorescence imaging, etc [61]. Among these, MRI, a medical imaging tool, is often chosen for its reliability, superior spatial clarity, outstanding contrast in softer tissues, high signal-to-noise ratio, and absence of harmful rays. MRI creates three-dimensional images of particular organs and tissues by employing radio waves along with a strong magnetic field [62–64].

In the last few decades, MNPs, including superparamagnetic iron oxide nanoparticles (SPIONs) and magnetic iron oxide nanoparticles (IONPs), have been widely studied to design theranostic agents for clinical applications. Numerous MNPs are undergoing clinical trials; many MNPs are FDA-approved and have reached the market [65–67]. To date, the European Commission (EC) and/or US FDA have approved five IONPs, including Feridex, Gastromark, Ferumoxytol, Resovist, and Sinerem, for use as MRI contrast agents for cancer diagnosis [68–70].

5.1.1 Nano-SMART (NCT04789486), gadolinium-based nanoparticles for diagnosis of pancreatic and lung cancer

A gadolinium-based nanoparticle, called Nano-SMART, is being examined in clinical trials for its potential to diagnose lung and pancreatic tumors in conjunction with stereotactic body radiotherapy (SBRT). This gadolinium-based nanoparticle improves the visibility of tumor tissues in MRI, allowing doctors to identify the size and severity of tumors more accurately. Additionally, it will make tumors more sensitive to radiation therapy such as SBRT. The clinical trial of Nano-SMART is recruiting study participants and is expected to be completed by 2027.

5.1.2 Iron oxide nanoparticle magnetic needle (NCT01411904) for detection of leukemia

Leukemia is a hematopoietic malignancy resulting from the overproduction of abnormal white blood cells (WBCs) [71]. Precisely measuring minimal residual disease (MRD) in these patients is essential for identifying prognosis and determining treatment approaches [39]. The University of New Mexico has designed a novel device, MagProbe, a magnetic needle made of IONPs. This needle was investigated in clinical studies to detect hematopoietic malignancies. The study's objective was to identify whether magnetic needles in the presence of MNPs could accurately detect MRD in patients with leukemia. MagProbe was withdrawn from clinical trials due to differences in MNPs obtained from the vendors.

5.1.3 Ferumoxtran-10 enhanced MRI (NCT04261777, NCT02751606, NCT00107484) for prostate, rectal, and breast cancer

Ferumoxtran-10, made of ultrasmall superparamagnetic iron oxide (USPIO) NPs, has gained interest as a valuable contrast agent for identifying metastases in lymph nodes using MRI in several types of cancer [72, 73]. The clinical trial of ferumoxtran-10 (NCT04261777) is in phase 3 and is evaluating the diagnostic potential of MRI with and without ferumoxtran-10. Nearly 296 men, with ages ranging from 47 to 83 years, suffering from prostate cancer participated in the clinical trial. Ferumoxtran-10 was intravenously administered to patients, followed by magnetic resonance (MR) lymphography of the pelvis after a day. Based on the results of MR lymphography, MRI-guided minimal extended pelvic lymph node dissection (PLND) or CT-guided biopsy was conducted. The researchers found that ferumoxtran-10 enhanced the MRI scans in nodal metastases outside the area of PLND in 41% of prostate cancer patients, highlighting the potential of ferumoxtran-10 as a contrast agent [41, 42]. Two hundred participants are already enrolled in a clinical trial, which is in the active stage and predicted to be finished by 2025.

Ferumoxtran-10, in combination with field MRI (7 T), is also undergoing clinical trials to detect lymph node metastases in breast and rectal cancer. Ferumoxtran-10 was administered to the affected area, and images were captured before and 24 h after contrast injection. Fifty-eight men and 19 women scheduled for surgical lymph node dissection with various types of cancer, including renal, bladder, endometrial, prostate, penile, breast, and ureteral cancers, were enrolled in the clinical trial. These patients underwent MRI scans before and 24–36 h after receiving ferumoxtran-10 (2.6 mg Fe/kg) intravenously. One hundred and sixty-nine lymph nodes were evaluated, and pre- and post-contrast MRI scans were compared. Histopathologic examination revealed that 114 of the 169 lymph nodes under investigation were malignant, while 55 were benign. This study demonstrated that images captured after ferumoxtran-10 administration could accurately characterize lymph nodes as benign or malignant, potentially leading to earlier and more precise cancer diagnosis and treatment [74].

5.1.4 Magnetic nanoparticles for determination of blood tumor cells (NCT04290923)

The oldest and most extensively studied technology is identifying circulating tumor cells (CTCs) with the help of MNPs in the bloodstream [75, 76]. The larger surface area-to-volume ratio and fast binding kinetics of MNPs make them ideal for forming bonds with CTCs. The MNPs used for this purpose are often decorated with antibodies, aptamers, or peptides to enhance the MNPs' specificity towards CTCs [76].

MNPs coated with anti-epithelial cell adhesion molecule (EpCAM) antibodies completed their clinical trial in 2022 (NCT04290923). These MNPs coated with anti-EpCAM were designed to interact with epithelial tumor cells. EpCAM is a tumor-associated biomarker expressed on epithelial cancer cells [77]. The objective of the research was to remove CTCs from the blood utilizing anti-EpCAM antibody as a marker. When MNPs coated in anti-EpCAM come into contact with the epithelial

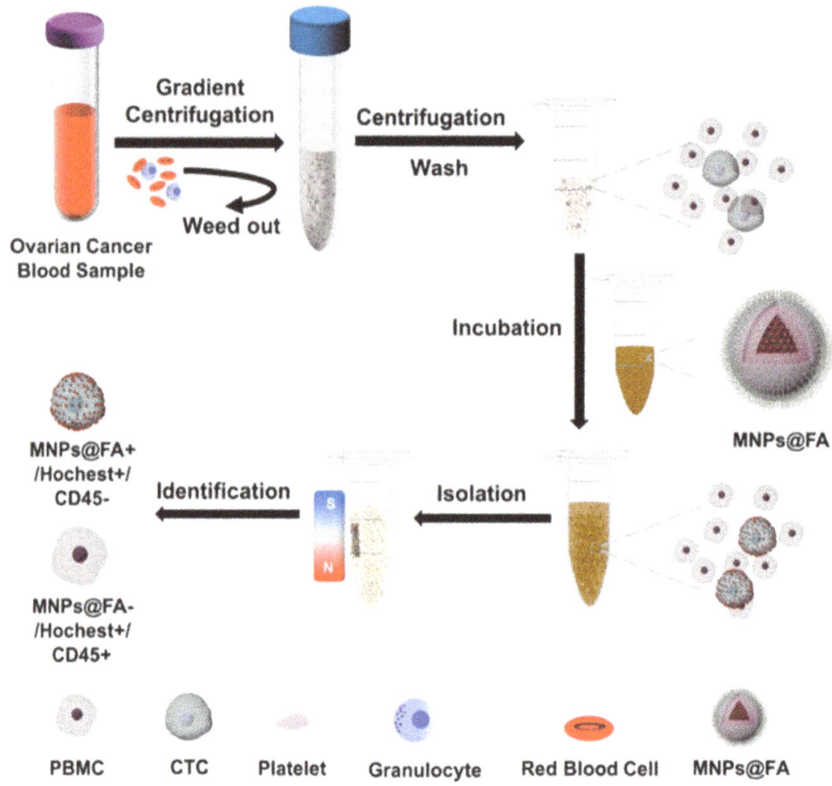

Figure 5.1. Schematic showing the process of CTC separation by MNPs conjugated with folic acid in a blood sample taken from a patient with ovarian cancer. Adapted from [78]. CC BY 4.0.

tumor cells, they form a magnetic complex that can be separated from the blood by applying a magnetic field. Nearly 100 patients with colon, prostate, pancreatic, and lung cancer were enrolled in this study. The researchers plan to extend their studies to nonsolid tumors such as lymphoma or leukemia, utilizing MNPs in combination with CD52, a protein expressed by lymphoma or leukemia cells. The trial's findings have not been published yet, but the completion of the study indicates the technology is safe for clinical use. MNP-based CTC detection could help doctors with earlier cancer diagnoses and assist them in planning accurate therapies. Pan *et al* functionalized MNPs with folic acid (FA@MNPs), which can separate CTCs obtained from patients with ovarian cancer (figure 5.1) [78]. FA@MNPs were added to blood samples collected from patients with ovarian cancer. FA@MNPs have the potential to bind to the tumor cells, and when a magnetic field is applied, the CTCs are separated from the blood sample.

5.1.5 Resovist (NCT00307866) as contrast enhancer in MRI for liver cancer

Liver cancer is a complex and heterogeneous disorder that has a poor prognosis [79, 80]. Ferumoxides (also known as Feridex or Endorem in the USA and Europe, respectively) and ferucarbotran (Resovist) are two SPIOs that the FDA has already approved as contrast-enhanced agents for MRI to detect liver cancer [81, 82]. It has been reported that SPIO-enhanced MRI provides more accurate detection of hepatic malignancy than unenhanced MRI [83, 84]. Resovist completed its multicenter clinical trial with 218 participants in 2005. The clinical study aimed to examine the effectiveness of Resovist-enhanced and unenhanced MRI and compare it with the contrast-enhanced dual-phase spiral CT obtained from patients with primary and secondary liver malignancies. The findings of the clinical trials have not yet been published publicly; however, these SPIOs are safe and usable, as they have completed their clinical trial and been approved by the FDA.

5.1.6 SPIO-enhanced MRI (NCT05359783) for sentinel node localization in breast cancer patients

The status of the sentinel lymph nodes (SLNs) serves as a prognostic biomarker in patients who have breast cancer [34, 85]. Currently, blue dye (BD) and technetium-99m (Tc-99m) are used to detect SLNs [86]. The aim of a current clinical trial of SPIO-enhanced MRI (NCT05359783) is to investigate the potential of SPIO to detect SLNs at ultralow doses. The clinical trial is in phase I/II and is in an active state. It has enrolled 50 females aged 18 years and older. The designed SPIO, called MagTrace, comprises an iron oxide NP core and a biocompatible hydrophilic coating. MagTrace will be administered to tumors through intradermal injection at a dose of 0.1 ml and injection will continue for seven days up to the day of surgery.

Several studies have been conducted comparing SPIO and Tc99 with or without BD to detect SLNs. Nakanishi *et al* studied the effectiveness of SPIO as a sole tracer in the preoperative setting. They carried out a cohort study in two hospitals, one using SPIO and the other using Tc99 [87]. They injected Tc99 on the day of surgery or one day before surgery. On the other hand, SPIO was injected one hour before surgery or before an operation took place in the outpatient clinic. Nearly 343 procedures were conducted in 338 patients with breast cancer. Tc99 was used in 159 procedures, and the SPIO NP-labeled tracer was used in 184 procedures. The rates of detection of Tc99 and SPIO were found to be 96.9% and 95.6%, respectively, showing no significant difference. These findings indicate that SPIO alone can act as a safe alternative, with results comparable to those of the standard dual technique used for SLN detection (figure 5.2).

5.2 Clinical trials of MNPs for therapeutic purposes in cancer

5.2.1 Magnetic particle thermoablation—retention in the prostate (NCT02033447)

The most prevalent kind of cancer diagnosis in men is prostate cancer, affecting one in 350 individuals [88, 89]. The current treatment options, such as surgery or radiotherapy, cause significant side effects and can also destroy the health of surrounding tissues, resulting in erectile dysfunction, urinary incontinence, discomfort, diarrhea, and sometimes rectal bleeding [90, 91]. Magnetic particle hyperthermia (MPH) is emerging as a promising and noninvasive technique for treating cancer utilizing heat energy [92, 93]. Initially, MNPs are administered to the tumor

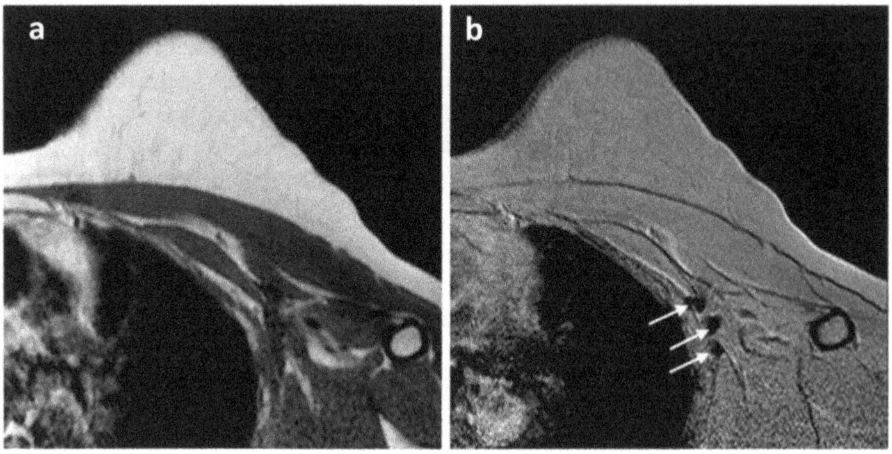

Figure 5.2. MRI scan of a patient with invasive ductal breast cancer. Panel (a) shows a T1-weighted image without visible SPIO accumulation in the lymph nodes, whereas panel (b) shows a T2*-weighted image with signal voids due to SPIO accumulation in three lymph nodes, providing an enhanced image. Adapted from [87]. CC BY 4.0.

site, followed by magnetic field exposure, which converts magnetic energy into heat energy. As tumor cells are sensitive to heat, they are destroyed without damaging healthy cells [93].

The primary objective of this study (NCT02033447) was to involve patients who had various amounts of MNPs injected into their prostate, after which the prostate was removed by radical surgery. Special scans were performed to confirm that the MNPs remained in the same place where they were injected, and then the patient was treated with magnetic thermoablation. This study completed its Early Phase 1 clinical trial in 2015, involving 18 participants who were undergoing radical cystoprostatectomy for bladder cancer or prostatectomy for prostate cancer (figure 5.3).

Jordan *et al* explored the effects of hyperthermia using MNPs in prostate cancer [95]. A 67-year-old patient who had undergone radiation therapy was chosen for the treatment. The MNPs were administered transperineally into the prostate region in sterile conditions under anesthesia, and transrectal US and fluoroscopy guidance were used to ensure that the MNPs were accurately placed. An alternating magnetic field was applied to heat the MNPs. Hyperthermic sessions were carried out for 60 min during the first and last six weeks. Following the initial and subsequent sessions of hyperthermia, CT images of the prostate were obtained to track the distribution of the MNPs and confirm the location of the thermometry probes inside the prostate. The findings indicated that MNPs can remain inside the prostate for more than one month, highlighting their potential for use in hyperthermia.

5.2.2 Adjuvant therapy of glioblastoma multiforme using MNPs (NCT06271421)

Glioblastoma multiforme (GBM) is one of the widely known primary brain tumors [51, 96, 97]. Surgical excision of the tumor is the main treatment option; however,

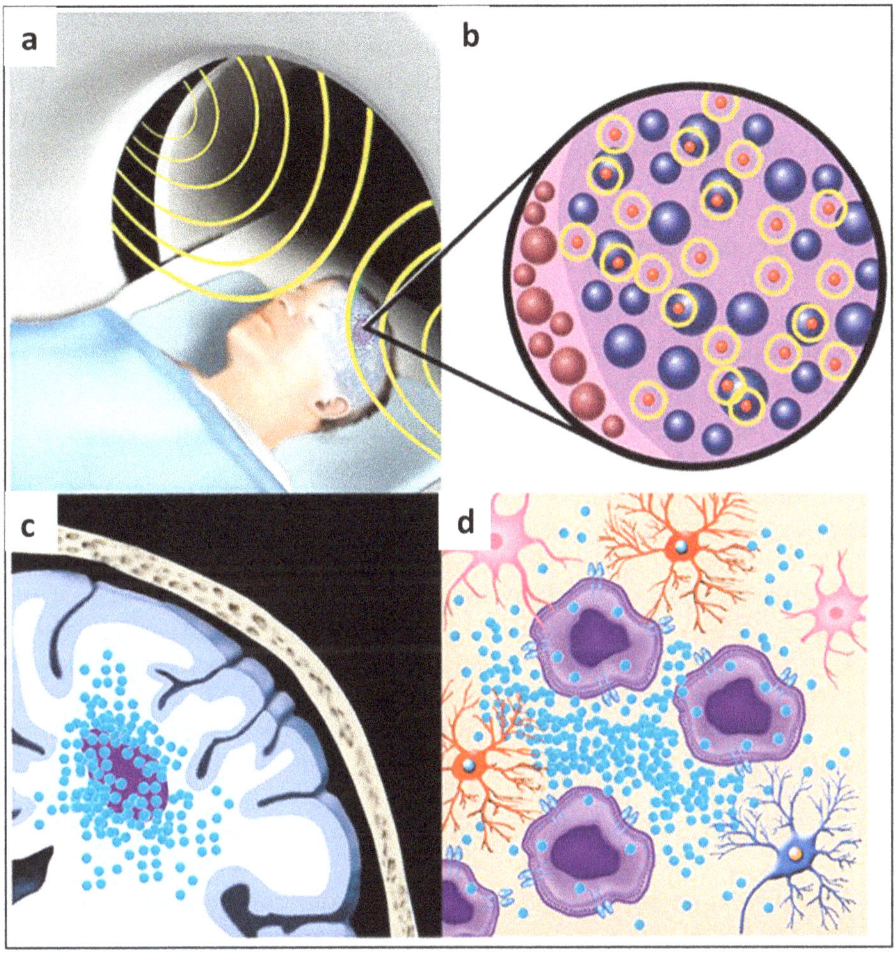

Figure 5.3. Following MNP implantation, a person with a brain tumor is treated via local hyperthermia. (a) To produce local hyperthermia in the tumor area, the patient is exposed to an alternating magnetic field (AMF) (yellow). (b) The thermotherapeutic effect is produced by the oscillation of the MNPs (yellow) inside and around the tumor cells. (c) A targeted therapeutic effect is produced by localized implantation of the MNPs inside and around the brain tumor. (d) Due to increased intracellular absorption of MNPs and sensitivity to temperature changes, brain tumor cells might be more vulnerable to the consequences of local hyperthermia. Adapted from [94]. CC BY 4.0.

since GBM affects the entire brain, complete resection is not feasible, so the use of adjuvant chemotherapy and/or radiation therapy is recommended by the Stupp protocol.

NanoTherm therapy involving cyclic hyperthermia in GBM patients is currently undergoing clinical trial, which is estimated to be completed by 2027. The study is recruiting participants for the clinical trial. The primary goal of the study is to assess the efficiency and tolerances of utilizing MNPs in cyclic hyperthermia as an adjuvant treatment in GBM patients, prolonging their survival rate and improving their quality of life. The literature indicates that such patients have an average overall survival of nine to twelve months [98]. According to research conducted by Maier-Hauff *et al*, patients receiving NanoTherm therapy following recurrence had a median survival time of 13.4 months, which was a significantly greater duration ($P < 0.01$) than those receiving Stupp protocol treatment (6.2 months). Following a first diagnosis of GBM, the average survival was also longer (23.2 versus 14.6 months). The implementation of NanoTherm therapy was credited for the improvement seen in both patient groups [98].

5.2.3 MR-L-SPION (NCT04682847), SPIONs (superparamagnetic iron oxide nanoparticles) for hepatocellular carcinomas

Patients with liver cancer are at greater risk of radiation-induced liver disease (RILD) and hepatic cirrhosis when undergoing SBRT [99, 100]. A clinical trial (NCT04682847) of MR-linac treatment combined with SPIONs (MR-L-SPIONs) is being investigated to overcome these challenges and improve the safety and effectiveness of SBRT for patients with hepatocellular carcinomas (HCCs). MR-L-SPION combines SPIONs, SBRT, and cellular magnetic resonance imaging (CMRI) with MR-linac treatment to identify both primary and metastatic hepatic malignancies. SPIONs will accumulate in the tumor region, enhancing its visibility in MRI. CMRI will determine the functional hepatic parenchyma that needs to be spared from exposure to over-threshold radiation when SBRT is administered. In this way, MR-L-SPION will substantially enhance diagnostic accuracy by determining the safe volume of functional liver tissue when planning SBRT administered by MR-linac and improve the safety of patients with preexisting liver damage. The MR-L-SPION trial is in the active stage, and 40 participants have been enrolled.

5.2.4 Chemotherapy with superparamagnetic iron oxide nanoparticles (NCT04316091) for management of osteosarcoma

Osteosarcoma, a primary aggressive bone tumor, mainly affects children and adolescents [101–103]. Although intensive chemotherapy and surgical resection combined have improved the survival rate from 51% to 75%, various adverse effects are seen to compromise the survival rate of patients.

In the current study, researchers have investigated the use of neoadjuvant chemotherapy and SPIONs with a spinning magnetic field (SMF) to permanently remove cancer cells and shrink tumors while preserving local structures and functions in patients who are unable to receive therapy for limb retention. Sixty osteosarcoma patients have been enrolled in the phase I clinical trial. The purpose of the study is to examine the safety, effectiveness, and tolerance of SPIONs/SMF in patients with osteosarcoma when used in conjunction with neoadjuvant chemotherapy. These patients will receive three intratumoral injections of SPIONs every other day, followed by two hours of SMF every two days for a month. Starting on day one, they will receive standard neoadjuvant chemotherapy. The sponsor believes that SPIONs/SMF will function synergistically with neoadjuvant chemotherapy to boost cancer cell killing, improve the effectiveness of neoadjuvant treatment with chemotherapy, and enhance the percentage of limb retention. After that, all patients will be subsequently followed up every two months for health evaluations to assess the status of malignancies until the end of the study.

5.2.5 NANO-RAD for treatment of multiple brain metastases (NCT02820454 and NCT03818386)

In radiation therapy, high-energy x-rays are utilized to disrupt cancer tissues [104–106]. It has been reported that AGuIX particles make tumor cells more sensitive to radiation and can be combined with radiotherapy to improve the effectiveness of radiation therapy [107]. The current NANO-RAD (NCT02820454) study aims to evaluate the tolerability, safety, and side effects of AGuIX combined with whole brain radiation therapy (WBRT) in patients suffering from multiple brain tumors.

In order to visualize the spatial distribution of AGuIX in brain tumors and surrounding healthy tissues, as well as to assess the contrast improvement in brain metastases, patients will receive a single intravenous injection of AGuIX on the first day of treatment. Two hours after the AGuIX injection, patients will undergo WBRT, which will continue for two weeks, five days a week. The NANO-RAD study completed its first-in-human Phase I trial in 2019 with 15 participants. The results of the trial have not been published yet [108]. After the successful completion of the phase 1 clinical trial, NANO-RAD is now in its phase 2 clinical trial (NCT03818386) and has enrolled nearly 100 participants. It is estimated that it will be completed by 2025.

5.2.6 NBTXR3 in addition to radiation therapy for cancer (NCT04484909, NCT01946867)

NBTXR3 consists of functionalized hafnium oxide nanoparticles that act as a radio enhancer, which enhances the absorption of ionizing radiation, leading to increased cancer cell death without causing any harm to nearby healthy cells [60, 109–112] Various clinical trials are being carried out using NBTXR3 in addition to radiation therapy as a treatment approach for numerous types of cancer, including liver, pancreatic, oral cavity, soft tissue, esophagus, lung cancer, etc [56, 58–60, 113, 114].

Bagley *et al* treated a 66-year-old man suffering from unresectable locally advanced pancreatic ductal adenocarcinoma using radiation therapy that was activated by NBTXR3 (NCT04484909). The patient was exposed to radiation after 12 days of NBTXR3 injections. The lesion size was radiographically stable, and the patient did not experience any treatment-related side effects.

A study conducted by Hoffmann *et al* is in a phase 1 clinical trial (NCT01946867). The main objective of this research is to examine the effectiveness of NBTXR3 in individuals with locally advanced head and neck cancer who are not suitable candidates for chemoradiation. Throughout the process of radiation therapy, NBTXR3 is observed to stay within the injected tumor without leaking into the healthy tissue surrounding it, highlighting antitumor effects.

5.3 Patents filed on magnetic MNPs for advanced cancer theranostics

Plenty of research has been carried out on magnetic-based systems containing MNPs due to their unique characteristics when applied in MRI, magnetic targeting, hyperthermia, and precise drug delivery and release. MNPs, specifically SPIONs, are explored in imaging techniques such as MRI as contrast enhancers to visualize cancerous tissues better. They are often conjugated with chemotherapeutic drugs to carry them to the target site and improve treatment effectiveness while minimizing side effects [11, 115, 116]. MNPs are frequently decorated using a broad range of components to strengthen their biological compatibility, transport therapeutic drugs, attach imaging agents, as well as offer functional groups for the conjugation of biological molecules that present receptor-mediated targeting for cancer [117–119]. Various patents have been filed describing innovative approaches utilizing MNPs to enhance theranostic efficacy against cancer. Some of the recently filed patents are listed in table 5.2.

5.3.1 MNPs for treating cancer (WO2019072885A1)

This patent, filed by INSERM (Institut National de la Santé et de la Recherche Médicale), relates to pharmaceutical compositions and methods for the treatment of cancer using MNPs that can generate magnetic intra-lysosomal hyperthermia (MILH). Researchers functionalized MNPs with ligands of receptors that are overexpressed in tumors. These MNPs were then administered to lysosomes of cancerous cells. MNPs can raise the temperature of the surrounding area even at low heating power [144, 145]. This rise in temperature causes lysosomal membrane permeabilization (LMP), an early event triggering apoptosis [146–149]. MNPs bind to the lysosome and release lysosomal hydrolases such as cathepsin B and cathepsin D into the cytosol, which breaks down the apoptosis-regulated proteins, causing mitochondrial outer membrane permeabilization (MOMP) and activation of apoptotic pathways [150–152].

Researchers at INSERM discovered that MILH causes cell death through a non-apoptotic signaling pathway that is dependent on caspase-1 and cathepsin B but does not involve apoptotic caspase-3 when subjected to an AMF. When exposed to LMP, the Fenton reaction in lysosomes produces reactive oxygen species (ROS), which causes lipid peroxidation of the lysosomal membrane. These findings provide a deeper understanding of the mechanism of cell death during MILH and will be useful in optimizing the approach from a therapeutic viewpoint.

5.3.2 Composite magnetic nanoparticle drug delivery system (US20120265001)

This application was granted to Wichita State University (WSU) in 2017. Researchers at WSU have developed a composite MNP (Fe_3O_4) drug delivery system that offers targeted and controlled release of chemotherapy at tumor sites. This system can be administered to a patient through various routes, including oral, pulmonary or inhalation, transmucosal, nasal, cardiovascular, colorectal,

Table 5.2. Selected recent patents filed for MNPs intended for use in cancer theranostics.

Sl. No,	Publication no.	Filing country	Filed by	Application	Issue/ Publication date	Status	References
1.	EP3960200A1	Europe	Politechnika Wrocławska	Active MNPs as a carrier of biologically active agents and drugs to treat cancers, including breast cancer	2022-03-02	Withdrawn	[120]
2.	US11324841B2	United States	Intron Biotechnology Inc.	Metal oxide nanoparticle contrast and drug delivery agent for cancer treatment	2021-01-14	Active	[121]
3.	US9952209B2	United States	University of Memphis Research Foundation	Photothermal therapy using iron oxide–gold core–shell nanoparticles	2018-04-24	Active	[122]
4.	US11077191B2	United States	Southeast Missouri State University	Destruction of cancer cells using smart nanostructures made of MNPs	2021-08-03	Active	[123]
5.	US10828414B2	United States	University of California	Magnetic filtration devices to purify blood flowing in a blood vessel	2018-02-15	Active	[124]
6.	CN107899013B	China	Zhengzhou University	Photodynamic therapy in combination with mesoporous manganese dioxide nanodrug loading system for the treatment of breast cancer	2020-01-14	Active	[125]
7.	JP2019536716A	Japan	Neo-Nanomedics, Inc.	IONPs doped with alkali metal or alkaline earth metal for hyperthermic treatment	2019-12-19	Active	[126]

(*Continued*)

Table 5.2. *(Continued)*

Sl. No,	Publication no.	Filing country	Filed by	Application	Issue/ Publication date	Status	References
8.	CN109953973A	China	Cai Xiaohui	Novel pH-sensitive magnetic targeted nanometer medicine-carried system to reduce the toxic side effects of chemotherapeutics when treating lymphoma	2019-07-02	Pending	[127]
9.	US11918315B2	United States	Pulse Therapeutics Inc.	Determination of structure and traversal of occlusions using magnetic particles	2024-03-05	Active	[128]
10.	CN109125742B	China	Zhenjiang First Peoples Hospital	IONPs in tumor targeted diagnosis and treatment	2021-08-24	Expired - Fee Related	[129]
11.	KR102527690B1	South Korea	NBS ST Co., Ltd	Photothermal MNPs to destroy targeted cancer cells	2023-05-02		[130]
12.	CN114521882B	China	Beihang University	Magnetic particle-based field-free line scanning imaging and field-free point positioning thermotherapy fusion device	2022-07-19	Active	[131]
13.	WO2020034696A1	WIPO (PCT)	Jiangsu Institute of Traditional Chinese Medicine	Superparamagnetic oxide nanoparticles as drug delivery system	2020-02-20		[132]
14.	CN106913885B	China	Ningbo Institute of Material Technology and Engineering of CAS	MNPs as high-quality MRI contrast agent	2020-05-08	Active	[133]

15.	KR102087825B1	South Korea	Wonkwang University Industry-Academic Cooperation Foundation	Magnetic-field- driven therapy device for cancer treatment			[134]
16.	US20180050218A1	United States	Nimd Ltd	Hyperthermic cancer treatment using ferromagnetic nanoparticles	2018-02-22	Abandoned	[135]
17.	CN109626439B	China	Ningbo Institute of Material Technology and Engineering of CAS	Metal-doped ferrite ($M_xFe_{3-x}O_4$) NPs as contrast agent in MRI	2024-05-07	Active	[136]
18.	CN112957467A	China	Ninth Peoples Hospital Shanghai Jiaotong University	Nano diagnosis and treatment agent made of superparamagnetic ferroferric oxide nanoparticles with a calcium carbonate layer coated on their surface	2021-06-15	Active	[137]
19.	US10179179B2	United States	Nano and Advanced Materials Institute Ltd	MNPs as a contrast agent in MRI	2019-01-15	Active	[138]
20.	CN109453395A	China	Suzhou Nagenuosi Biological Technology Co Ltd	Monodisperse fluorescent MNPs for diagnosis and treatment of cancer	2019-03-12	Pending	[139]
21.	RU2633918C2	Russia	Limited Liability Company 'Farmag'	Magnetic hyperthermic treatment of malignant neoplasms using Zn-substituted MNPs	2017-12-28		[140]
22.	US9555136B2	United States	University of Washington Center for Commercialization	Polymer-coated iron oxide MNPs for cancer theranostics	2017-01-31	Active	[141]
23.	US20210300754A1	United States	Lyubov Ostrovska	Tumor identification along with targeted hyperthermia	2021-09-30	Abandoned	[142]
24.	US20210220480A1	United States	Gholam A. Peyman	Cancer treatment and imaging	2021-07-22	Pending	[143]

parenteral, or intraosseous methods. Alternatively, it can be delivered via a catheter to the cancerous tumor or inflammation site. A magnet attracts the magnetic composite nanoparticles to the affected region, and the MNPs are taken into the affected area by the biological targeting component. When the biodegradable polymer degrades or breaks down, the drug is released in a controlled, time-dependent manner into the targeted area. This novel drug delivery system may be used to treat or prevent cancer, disease, or other conditions.

5.3.3 A kind of preparation method for dual-target magnetic nanoparticles for treating liver cancer (CN109701039A)

Zhejiang University (ZJU) filed this application in 2019 related to a preparation method of dual-target MNPs for liver cancer. HCC is the fifth most common type of cancer worldwide [153, 154]. Researchers at ZJU developed a dual-target MNP based on superparamagnetic nanoparticle ferrosoferric oxide (Fe_3O_4) for liver cancer. They modified the surface of Fe_3O_4 by attaching an anti-alpha-fetoprotein (AFP) and anti-CD34 antibody complex to it, forming SPIO-PEG-BsAb. This functionalized SPIO-PEG-BsAb can act as a dynamic tracer for liver cancer cells and liver cancer neovascular endothelial cells in MRI. SPIO-PEG-BsAb not only functions as a dynamic tracer in living bodies but can also detect tumor neovascular blood vessels at the molecular level. This dynamic evaluation of SPIO-PEG-BsAb provides new approaches and ways for planning appropriate treatment strategies for cancer.

5.3.4 Preparation and application of an ultrahigh-field magnetic resonance contrast enhancer (CN112274657B)

This is another application granted to ZJU in 2022 that relates to an ultrahigh-field MR contrast agent, which comprises MNPs 5 nm in size that can be selected from a choice of sodium gadolinium tetrafluoride nanoparticles, manganese oxide nanoparticles, cobalt oxide nanoparticles, or IONPs. This invention aims to provide an ultrahigh-field MR contrast agent that can be used for accurately evaluating the permeability of tumor vessels and has high sensitivity.

5.3.5 Preparation and application of magnetic nanodrug carrier (CN112870387A)

This patent application relates to the design of a magnetic nanodrug carrier based on SPIONs that carries the SP94 targeting peptide and a coupling product of a small interfering RNA (siRNA). This invention proves that the nanodrug carrier effectively provides good biocompatibility, stability, targeting properties, low immunogenicity, high gene transfection efficiency, and drug release properties. These properties make magnetic nanodrug carriers a promising option for use in the preparation of cancer gene therapy drugs. This application was granted to Sun Yat-Sen Memorial Hospital, Sun Yat-Sen University in 2023 and is active.

5.3.6 Imaging device for in vivo nondestructive detection of skin cancer and application method thereof (CN118370528A)

Recently, researchers from Suzhou Institute of Higher Studies at the University of Science And Technology Of China have applied for a patent for an imaging device that can detect skin cancer by utilizing superparamagnetic nanoparticles to identify lesioned tissues in the skin. If malignancies of the skin fail to be identified early, skin cancers are predicted to increase significantly in the next 20 years [155, 156]. Squamous cell cancer, basal cell carcinoma, aggressive melanoma, and eczematoid malignancies are the main forms of primary skin cancer [157, 158]. Focusing on the early diagnosis of skin cancer, particularly malignant melanoma with the highest mortality rate, can significantly improve detection methods. The currently available imaging methods include skin optical coherence tomography (OCT), skin CT, dermatoscopy, ultrasonic B-scanning, skin PA imaging, local CT/MRI/PET-CT, whole-body and skin terahertz imaging, etc [159–161] Although existing techniques can diagnose and identify tissue structure lesions, they lack molecular-level diagnostic capability. This invention provides a molecular-pathology-level detection device suitable for *in vivo*, nondestructive use in skin tissue. It targets and marks pathological tissue in the skin using superparamagnetic nanoparticles. The device utilizes high-concentration ensemble nitrogen vacancy (NV) color centers in diamond to measure the magnetic signals produced by these nanoparticles. This approach enables accurate and sensitive detection of skin cancer, thereby providing a new technical means for basic research and clinical diagnosis of skin tumor diseases.

5.3.7 Method for tumor detection and targeted hyperthermia (US20210300754A1)

This US patent, filed by Lyubov Ostrovska in 2021, relates to stem cells that are loaded with bifunctional MNPs (nanoparticle-loaded stem cells (NLSCs)) for MR-guided hyperthermia. The MNPs in the NLSCs are biocompatible and do not interfere with the proliferation and differentiation of the stem cells. It has been reported that circulating stem cells are home to tumors and metastases and participate in neovascularization in growing tumors [162–164]. The NLSCs described in this patent application enable the tracking of the tissue distribution of infused stem cells and the selective heating of targeted tissues with an AMF. By applying hyperthermia to hypoxic regions of tumors, NLSCs can make those areas more sensitive to future treatments, thereby delivering therapy to tumor regions that are most resistant to treatment. Either direct cell death occurs when diseased tissue is heated, or the tumor becomes more vulnerable to chemotherapy and/or radiation therapy. Because the targeted hyperthermia offered by this invention has fewer side effects and can be used in conjunction with traditional treatment modalities to greatly increase their efficacy, it has clinical potential. These NLSCs can be used to remove mis-injected stem cells, track and heat cells in stem cell research, and facilitate MR image-guided hyperthermia in oncology.

References and further reading

[1] Klement R J 2024 Cancer as a global health crisis with deep evolutionary roots *Global Trans.* **6** 45–65

[2] Gosse R A, Msengi E A, Chona E Z and Ambikile J S 2024 Experiences of caring for women with cervical cancer: a qualitative study among male partners in Dar es Salaam, Tanzania *Health Exp.* **27** e14038

[3] Katib Y and Mulla N 2024 Epidemiological and clinical characteristics of lung cancer in Saudi Arabia: a retrospective study in single oncology center *Oncol. Res.* **32** 1803–9

[4] Spratt D E, Shore N, Sartor O, Rathkopf D and Olivier K 2021 Treating the patient and not just the cancer: therapeutic burden in prostate cancer *Prostate Cancer Prostatic Dis.* **24** 647–61

[5] Sung H, Ferlay J, Siegel R L, Laversanne M, Soerjomataram I, Jemal A and Bray F 2021 Global cancer statistics 2020: GLOBOCAN estimates of incidence and mortality worldwide for 36 cancers in 185 countries *CA: Cancer J. Clin.* **71** 209–49

[6] Ferlay J, Colombet M, Soerjomataram I, Mathers C, Parkin D M, Piñeros M, Znaor A and Bray F 2019 Estimating the global cancer incidence and mortality in 2018: GLOBOCAN sources and methods *Int. J. Cancer* **144** 1941–53

[7] Karvelas E G, Lampropoulos N, Benos L, Karakasidis T and Sarris I E 2021 On the magnetic aggregation of Fe_3O_4 nanoparticles *Comput. Methods Programs Biomed.* **198** 105778

[8] Shi J, Kantoff P W, Wooster R and Farokhzad O C 2017 Cancer nanomedicine: progress, challenges and opportunities *Nat. Rev. Cancer* **17** 20–37

[9] Ventola C L 2017 Progress in nanomedicine: approved and investigational nanodrugs *Pharm. Therap.* **42** 742

[10] Li X, Li W, Wang M and Liao Z 2021 Magnetic nanoparticles for cancer theranostics: advances and prospects *J. Control. Release* **335** 437–48

[11] Farzin A, Etesami S A, Quint J, Memic A and Tamayol A 2020 Magnetic nanoparticles in cancer therapy and diagnosis *Adv. Healthcare Mater.* **9** 1901058

[12] Wu M and Huang S 2017 Magnetic nanoparticles in cancer diagnosis, drug delivery and treatment *Mol. Clin. Oncol.* **7** 738–46

[13] Meng Y Q, Shi Y N, Zhu Y P, Liu Y Q, Gu L W, Liu D D, Ma A, Xia F, Guo Q Y and Xu C C 2024 Recent trends in preparation and biomedical applications of iron oxide nanoparticles *J. Nanobiotechnol.* **22** 24

[14] Nuzhina J V, Shtil A A, Prilepskii A Y and Vinogradov V V 2019 Preclinical evaluation and clinical translation of magnetite-based nanomedicines *J. Drug Deliv. Sci. Technol.* **54** 101282

[15] Singh A and Sahoo S K 2014 Magnetic nanoparticles: a novel platform for cancer theranostics *Drug Discov. Today* **19** 474–81

[16] Laurent S, Forge D, Port M, Roch A, Robic C, Vander Elst L and Muller R N 2008 Magnetic iron oxide nanoparticles: synthesis, stabilization, vectorization, physicochemical characterizations, and biological applications *Chem. Rev.* **108** 2064–110

[17] Khizar S, Elkalla E, Zine N, Jaffrezic-Renault N, Errachid A and Elaissari A 2023 Magnetic nanoparticles: multifunctional tool for cancer therapy *Exp. Opin. Drug Deliv.* **20** 189–204

[18] Prijic S and Sersa G 2011 Magnetic nanoparticles as targeted delivery systems in oncology *Radiol. Oncol.* **45** 1–16

[19] Chowdhury P, Roberts A M, Khan S, Hafeez B B, Chauhan S C, Jaggi M and Yallapu M M 2017 Magnetic nanoformulations for prostate cancer *Drug Discov. Today* **22** 1233–41
[20] Huang Y, Hsu J C, Koo H and Cormode D P 2022 Repurposing ferumoxytol: diagnostic and therapeutic applications of an FDA-approved nanoparticle *Theranostics* **12** 796
[21] Alromi D A, Madani S Y and Seifalian A 2021 Emerging application of magnetic nanoparticles for diagnosis and treatment of cancer *Polymers* **13** 4146
[22] Moros M, Idiago-López J, Asín L, Moreno-Antolín E, Beola L, Grazú V, Fratila R M, Gutiérrez L and de la Fuente J M 2019 Triggering antitumoural drug release and gene expression by magnetic hyperthermia *Adv. Drug Deliv. Rev.* **138** 326–43
[23] Baghban R, Afarid M, Soleymani J and Rahimi M 2021 Were magnetic materials useful in cancer therapy? *Biomed. Pharmacother.* **144** 112321
[24] Johannsen M, Thiesen B, Wust P and Jordan A 2010 Magnetic nanoparticle hyperthermia for prostate cancer *Int. J. Hyperth.* **26** 790–5
[25] Cristofanilli M, Budd G T, Ellis M J, Stopeck A, Matera J, Miller M C, Reuben J M, Doyle G V, Allard W J and Terstappen L W 2004 Circulating tumor cells, disease progression, and survival in metastatic breast cancer *New Engl. J. Med.* **351** 781–91
[26] Herrmann I K, Bernabei R E, Urner M, Grass R N, Beck-Schimmer B and Stark W J 2011 Device for continuous extracorporeal blood purification using target-specific metal nanomagnets *Nephrol. Dial. Transpl.* **26** 2948–54
[27] Herrmann I K, Schlegel A, Graf R, Schumacher C M, Senn N, Hasler M, Gschwind S, Hirt A-M, Günther D and Clavien P-A 2013 Nanomagnet-based removal of lead and digoxin from living rats *Nanoscale* **5** 8718–23
[28] Fisher C S, Margenthaler J A, Hunt K K and Schwartz T 2020 The landmark series: axillary management in breast cancer *Ann. Surg. Oncol.* **27** 724–9
[29] Racz J M and Caudle A S 2019 Sentinel node lymph node surgery after neoadjuvant therapy: principles and techniques *Ann. Surg. Oncol.* **26** 3040–5
[30] Greenwood H I, Wong J M, Mukhtar R A, Alvarado M D and Price E R 2019 Feasibility of magnetic seeds for preoperative localization of axillary lymph nodes in breast cancer treatment *Am. J. Roentgenol.* **213** 953–7
[31] Karakatsanis A, Hersi A-F, Pistiolis L, Olofsson Bagge R, Lykoudis P, Eriksson S, Wärnberg F, Nagy G, Mohammed I and Sundqvist M 2019 Effect of preoperative injection of superparamagnetic iron oxide particles on rates of sentinel lymph node dissection in women undergoing surgery for ductal carcinoma *in situ* (SentiNot study) *J. Br. Surg.* **106** 720–8
[32] Pantiora E, Eriksson S, Wärnberg F and Karakatsanis A 2024 Magnetically guided surgery after primary systemic therapy for breast cancer: implications for enhanced axillary mapping *Br. J. Surg.* **111** znae008
[33] Karakatsanis A, Eriksson S, Pistiolis L, Olofsson Bagge R, Nagy G, Man V *et al* 2023 Delayed sentinel lymph node dissection in patients with a preoperative diagnosis of ductal cancer *in situ* by preoperative injection with superparamagnetic iron oxide (SPIO) nanoparticles: the SentiNot study *Ann. Surg. Oncol.* **30** 4064–72
[34] Waanders S, Visscher M, Wildeboer R, Oderkerk T, Krooshoop H and Ten Haken B 2016 A handheld SPIO-based sentinel lymph node mapping device using differential magnetometry *Phys. Med. Biol.* **61** 8120
[35] Karakatsanis A, Daskalakis K, Stålberg P, Olofsson H, Andersson Y, Eriksson S, Bergkvist L and Wärnberg F 2017 Superparamagnetic iron oxide nanoparticles as the

sole method for sentinel node biopsy detection in patients with breast cancer *J. Br. Surg.* **104** 1675–85

[36] Karakatsanis A, Christiansen P M, Fischer L, Hedin C, Pistioli L, Sund M, Rasmussen N R, Jørnsgård H, Tegnelius D and Eriksson S 2016 The Nordic SentiMag trial: a comparison of super paramagnetic iron oxide (SPIO) nanoparticles versus Tc 99 and patent blue in the detection of sentinel node (SN) in patients with breast cancer and a meta-analysis of earlier studies *Breast Cancer Res. Treat.* **157** 281–94

[37] Jazrawi A, Pantiora E, Abdsaleh S, Bacovia D V, Eriksson S, Leonhardt H, Wärnberg F and Karakatsanis A 2021 Magnetic-guided axillary ultrasound (MagUS) sentinel lymph node biopsy and mapping in patients with early breast cancer. a phase 2, single-arm prospective clinical trial *Cancers* **13** 4285

[38] Elhalawani H, Awan M J, Ding Y, Mohamed A S, Elsayes A K, Abu-Gheida I, Wang J, Hazle J, Gunn G B and Lai S Y 2020 Data from a terminated study on iron oxide nanoparticle magnetic resonance imaging for head and neck tumors *Sci. Data* **7** 63

[39] Jaetao J E, Butler K S, Adolphi N L, Lovato D M, Bryant H C, Rabinowitz I, Winter S S, Tessier T E, Hathaway H J and Bergemann C 2009 Enhanced leukemia cell detection using a novel magnetic needle and nanoparticles *Cancer Res.* **69** 8310–6

[40] Burkoň P, Trna J, Slávik M, Němeček R, Kazda T, Pospíšil P, Dastych M, Eid M, Novotný I and Procházka T 2022 Stereotactic Body Radiotherapy (SBRT) of pancreatic cancer—a critical review and practical consideration *Biomedicines* **10** 2480

[41] Heesakkers R A, Jager G J, Hovels A M, de Hoop B, van den Bosch H C, Raat F, Witjes J A, Mulders P F, van der Kaa C H and Barentsz J O 2009 Prostate cancer: detection of lymph node metastases outside the routine surgical area with ferumoxtran-10–enhanced MR imaging *Radiology* **251** 408–14

[42] Heesakkers R A, Hövels A M, Jager G J, van den Bosch H C, Witjes J A, Raat H P, Severens J L, Adang E M, van der Kaa C H and Fütterer J J 2008 MRI with a lymph-node-specific contrast agent as an alternative to CT scan and lymph-node dissection in patients with prostate cancer: a prospective multicohort study *Lancet Oncol.* **9** 850–6

[43] Harisinghani M G, Barentsz J, Hahn P F, Deserno W M, Tabatabaei S, van de Kaa C H, de la Rosette J and Weissleder R 2003 Noninvasive detection of clinically occult lymph-node metastases in prostate cancer *New Engl. J. Med.* **348** 2491–9

[44] D'Amico A V, Whittington R, Malkowicz S B, Schultz D, Blank K, Broderick G A, Tomaszewski J E, Renshaw A A, Kaplan I and Beard C J 1998 Biochemical outcome after radical prostatectomy, external beam radiation therapy, or interstitial radiation therapy for clinically localized prostate cancer *JAMA* **280** 969–74

[45] Verry C, Dufort S, Villa J, Gavard M, Iriart C, Grand S, Charles J, Chovelon B, Cracowski J-L and Quesada J-L 2021 Theranostic AGuIX nanoparticles as radiosensitizer: a phase I, dose-escalation study in patients with multiple brain metastases (NANO-RAD trial) *Radiother. Oncol.* **160** 159–65

[46] Le Duc G, Miladi I, Alric C, Mowat P, Bräuer-Krisch E, Bouchet A, Khalil E, Billotey C, Janier M and Lux F 2011 Toward an image-guided microbeam radiation therapy using gadolinium-based nanoparticles *ACS Nano* **5** 9566–74

[47] Lux F, Tran V L, Thomas E, Dufort S, Rossetti F, Martini M, Truillet C, Doussineau T, Bort G and Denat F 2019 AGuIX® from bench to bedside—transfer of an ultrasmall theranostic gadolinium-based nanoparticle to clinical medicine *Br. J. Radiol.* **92** 20180365

[48] Verry C, Dufort S, Barbier E L, Montigon O, Peoc'h M, Chartier P, Lux F, Balosso J, Tillement O and Sancey L 2016 MRI-guided clinical 6-MV radiosensitization of glioma using a unique gadolinium-based nanoparticles injection *Nanomedicine* **11** 2405–17

[49] Thivat E, Casile M, Moreau J, Molnar I, Dufort S, Seddik K, Le Duc G, De Beaumont O, Loeffler M and Durando X 2023 Phase I/II study testing the combination of AGuIX nanoparticles with radiochemotherapy and concomitant temozolomide in patients with newly diagnosed glioblastoma (NANO-GBM trial protocol) *BMC Cancer* **23** 344

[50] Robinson M J and Davis E J 2024 Neoadjuvant chemotherapy for adults with osteogenic sarcoma *Curr. Treatm. Opt. Oncol.* **25** 1366–73

[51] Stupp R, Taillibert S, Kanner A, Read W, Steinberg D M, Lhermitte B, Toms S, Idbaih A, Ahluwalia M S and Fink K 2017 Effect of tumor-treating fields plus maintenance temozolomide vs maintenance temozolomide alone on survival in patients with glioblastoma: a randomized clinical trial *JAMA* **318** 2306–16

[52] Gupta R and Sharma D 2019 Evolution of magnetic hyperthermia for glioblastoma multiforme therapy *ACS Chem. Neurosci.* **10** 1157–72

[53] Grauer O, Jaber M, Hess K, Weckesser M, Schwindt W, Maring S, Wölfer J and Stummer W 2019 Combined intracavitary thermotherapy with iron oxide nanoparticles and radiotherapy as local treatment modality in recurrent glioblastoma patients *J. Neuro-Oncol.* **141** 83–94

[54] Boroon M P, Ayani M-B and Bazaz S R 2018 Estimation of the optimum number and location of nanoparticle injections and the specific loss power for ideal hyperthermia *J. Therm. Biol* **72** 127–36

[55] Pinel S, Thomas N, Boura C and Barberi-Heyob M 2019 Approaches to physical stimulation of metallic nanoparticles for glioblastoma treatment *Adv. Drug Deliv. Rev.* **138** 344–57

[56] Hoffmann C, Calugaru V, Borcoman E, Moreno V, Calvo E, Liem X, Salas S, Doger B, Jouffroy T and Mirabel X 2021 Phase I dose-escalation study of NBTXR3 activated by intensity-modulated radiation therapy in elderly patients with locally advanced squamous cell carcinoma of the oral cavity or oropharynx *Eur. J. Cancer* **146** 135–44

[57] Maury P, Mondini M, Chargari C, Darricau A, Shahin M, Ammari S, Bockel S, Genestie C, Wu T-D and Lux F 2023 Clinical transfer of AGuIX®-based radiation treatments for locally advanced cervical cancer: MR quantification and *in vitro* insights in the NANOCOL clinical trial framework *Nanomed. Nanotechnol. Biol. Med.* **50** 102676

[58] Shen C, Frakes J, Niu J, Weiss J, Caudell J, Seiwert T, Said P, Guedj M, Tyan P and Vivar O 2022 684 NBTXR3 activated by radiotherapy in combination with nivolumab or pembrolizumab in patients with advanced cancers: results from an ongoing dose escalation phase I trial (Study 1100) *J. immunother. cancer* **10** A714

[59] Bonvalot S, Rutkowski P L, Thariat J, Carrère S, Ducassou A, Sunyach M-P, Agoston P, Hong A, Mervoyer A and Rastrelli M 2019 NBTXR3, a first-in-class radioenhancer hafnium oxide nanoparticle, plus radiotherapy versus radiotherapy alone in patients with locally advanced soft-tissue sarcoma (Act. In. Sarc): a multicentre, phase 2–3, randomised, controlled trial *Lancet Oncol.* **20** 1148–59

[60] Bagley A F, Ludmir E B, Maitra A, Minsky B D, Smith G L, Das P, Koong A C, Holliday E B, Taniguchi C M and Katz M H 2022 NBTXR3, a first-in-class radioenhancer for pancreatic ductal adenocarcinoma: report of first patient experience *Clin. Transl. Radiat. Oncol.* **33** 66–9

[61] European Society of Radiology (ESR) 2011 Medical imaging in personalised medicine: a white paper of the research committee of the European Society of Radiology (ESR) *Insights Imaging* **2** 621–30
[62] Rahman M 2023 Magnetic resonance imaging and iron-oxide nanoparticles in the era of personalized medicine *Nanotheranostics* **7** 424
[63] Cruz L J, Que I, Aswendt M, Chan A, Hoehn M and Löwik C 2016 Targeted nanoparticles for the non-invasive detection of traumatic brain injury by optical imaging and fluorine magnetic resonance imaging *Nano Res.* **9** 1276–89
[64] Lapusan R, Borlan R and Focsan M 2024 Advancing MRI with magnetic nanoparticles: a comprehensive review of translational research and clinical trials *Nanoscale Adv.* **6** 2234–59
[65] Fu G, Zhu L, Yang K, Zhuang R, Xie J and Zhang F 2016 Diffusion-weighted magnetic resonance imaging for therapy response monitoring and early treatment prediction of photothermal therapy *ACS Appl. Mater. Interfaces* **8** 5137–47
[66] Zhang F, Huang X, Zhu L, Guo N, Niu G, Swierczewska M, Lee S, Xu H, Wang A Y and Mohamedali K A 2012 Noninvasive monitoring of orthotopic glioblastoma therapy response using RGD-conjugated iron oxide nanoparticles *Biomaterials* **33** 5414–22
[67] Wang G, Zhang F, Tian R, Zhang L, Fu G, Yang L and Zhu L 2016 Nanotubes-embedded indocyanine green–hyaluronic acid nanoparticles for photoacoustic-imaging-guided phototherapy *ACS Appl. Mater. Interfaces* **8** 5608–17
[68] Huang J, Li Y, Orza A, Lu Q, Guo P, Wang L, Yang L and Mao H 2016 Magnetic nanoparticle facilitated drug delivery for cancer therapy with targeted and image-guided approaches *Adv. Funct. Mater.* **26** 3818–36
[69] Laurent S, Boutry S, Mahieu I, Elst L V and Muller R 2009 Iron oxide based MR contrast agents: from chemistry to cell labeling *Curr. Med. Chem.* **16** 4712–27
[70] Zhu L, Zhou Z, Mao H and Yang L 2017 Magnetic nanoparticles for precision oncology: theranostic magnetic iron oxide nanoparticles for image-guided and targeted cancer therapy *Nanomedicine* **12** 73–87
[71] Wang W, An J, Zhao R, Geng X, Jiang W, Yan X and Jiang B 2024 Nanozymes: a new approach for leukemia therapy *J. Mater. Chem.* B **12** 2459–70
[72] Stijns R C, Philips B W, Nagtegaal I D, Polat F, de Wilt J H, Wauters C A, Zamecnik P, Fütterer J J and Scheenen T W 2021 USPIO-enhanced MRI of lymph nodes in rectal cancer: a node-to-node comparison with histopathology *Eur. J. Radiol.* **138** 109636
[73] Fortuin A S, Brüggemann R, van der Linden J, Panfilov I, Israël B, Scheenen T W and Barentsz J O 2018 Ultra-small superparamagnetic iron oxides for metastatic lymph node detection: back on the block *Wiley Interdiscip. Rev. Nanomed. Nanobiotechnol.* **10** e1471
[74] Harisinghani M G, Saksena M A, Hahn P F, King B, Kim J, Torabi M T and Weissleder R 2006 Ferumoxtran-10-enhanced MR lymphangiography: does contrast-enhanced imaging alone suffice for accurate lymph node characterization? *Am. J. Roentgenol.* **186** 144–8
[75] Yun Y, Kim S, Lee S-N, Cho H-Y and Choi J-W 2024 Nanomaterial-based detection of circulating tumor cells and circulating cancer stem cells for cancer immunotherapy *Nano Converg.* **11** 1–27
[76] Bashir S, Amn Zia M, Shoukat M, Kaleem I and Bashir S 2024 Nanoparticles as a novel key driver for the isolation and detection of circulating tumour cells *Sci. Rep.* **14** 22580
[77] Hosono H, Ohishi T, Takei J, Asano T, Sayama Y, Kawada M, Kaneko M K and Kato Y 2020 The anti-epithelial cell adhesion molecule (EpCAM) monoclonal antibody EpMab-16 exerts antitumor activity in a mouse model of colorectal adenocarcinoma *Oncol. Lett.* **20** 383

[78] Pan Y, Wang Z, Ma J, Zhou T, Wu Z, Ding P, Sun N, Liu L, Pei R and Zhu W 2022 Folic acid-modified fluorescent-magnetic nanoparticles for efficient isolation and identification of circulating tumor cells in ovarian cancer *Biosensors* **12** 184
[79] Mahmoud A and Takaoka E 2025 An enhanced machine learning approach with stacking ensemble learner for accurate liver cancer diagnosis using feature selection and gene expression data *Healthc. Anal.* **7** 100373
[80] Fu J and Wang H 2018 Precision diagnosis and treatment of liver cancer in China *Cancer Lett.* **412** 283–8
[81] Wang Y-X J 2011 Superparamagnetic iron oxide based MRI contrast agents: Current status of clinical application *Quant. Imag. Med. Surg.* **1** 35
[82] Reimer P and Balzer T 2003 Ferucarbotran (Resovist): a new clinically approved RES-specific contrast agent for contrast-enhanced MRI of the liver: properties, clinical development, and applications *Eur. Radiol.* **13** 1266–76
[83] Li Y-W, Chen Z-G, Wang J-C and Zhang Z-M 2015 Superparamagnetic iron oxide-enhanced magnetic resonance imaging for focal hepatic lesions: systematic review and meta-analysis *World J. Gastroenterol.: WJG* **21** 4334
[84] 2016 Iron oxide *Meyler's Side Effects of Drugs* 16th edn ed J K Aronson (Amsterdam: Elsevier) 321–2
[85] Marmé F, Krieghoff-Henning E, Gerber B, Schmitt M, Zahm D-M, Bauerschlag D, Forstbauer H, Hildebrandt G, Ataseven B and Brodkorb T 2023 Deep learning to predict breast cancer sentinel lymph node status on INSEMA histological images *Eur. J. Cancer* **195** 113390
[86] Mirzaei N, Katsarelias D, Zaar P, Jalnefjord O, Johansson I, Leonhardt H, Wärnberg F and Bagge R O 2022 Sentinel lymph node localization and staging with a low-dose of superparamagnetic iron oxide (SPIO) enhanced MRI and magnetometer in patients with cutaneous melanoma of the extremity-The MAGMEN feasibility study *Eur. J. Surg. Oncol.* **48** 326–32
[87] Christenhusz A, Pouw J J, Simonis F F, Douek M, Ahmed M, Klaase J M, Dassen A E, Klazen C A, van der Schaaf M C and Ten Haken B 2022 Breast MRI in patients after breast conserving surgery with sentinel node procedure using a superparamagnetic tracer *Eur. Radiol. Exp.* **6** 3
[88] Bray F, Ferlay J, Soerjomataram I, Siegel R L, Torre L A and Jemal A 2018 Global cancer statistics 2018: GLOBOCAN estimates of incidence and mortality worldwide for 36 cancers in 185 countries *CA: Cancer J. Clin.* **68** 394–424
[89] Rawla P 2019 Epidemiology of prostate cancer *World J. Oncol.* **10** 63
[90] Michaelson M D, Cotter S E, Gargollo P C, Zietman A L, Dahl D M and Smith M R 2008 Management of complications of prostate cancer treatment *CA Cancer J Clin.* **58** 196–213
[91] Mahmood J, Shamah A A, Creed T M, Pavlovic R, Matsui H, Kimura M, Molitoris J, Shukla H, Jackson I and Vujaskovic Z 2016 Radiation-induced erectile dysfunction: Recent advances and future directions *Adv. Radiat. Onco.* **1** 161–9
[92] Zargar F A, Khanday M A and Ashraf M 2023 A mathematical study of nanoparticle aided hyperthermia treatment of hepatic cancer using magnetite nanoparticles under alternating and rotating magnetic fields *Int. J. Nonlinear Anal. Appl.* **14** 2301–12
[93] Zargar F, Bhat H A, Zargar M A and Malik S 2024 Magnetic nanoparticles in cancer thermotherapy: a mathematical approach to optimal treatment design *MatSci Express* **1** 116–24

[94] Mahmoudi K and Hadjipanayis C G 2014 The Application of Magnetic Nanoparticles for the Treatment of Brain Tumors *Front. Chem* **2** 109

[95] Johannsen M, Gneveckow U, Eckelt L, Feussner A, Waldöfner N, Scholz R, Deger S, Wust P, Loening S and Jordan A 2005 Clinical hyperthermia of prostate cancer using magnetic nanoparticles: presentation of a new interstitial technique *Int. J. Hyperth.* **21** 637–47

[96] Wu W, Klockow J L, Zhang M, Lafortune F, Chang E, Jin L, Wu Y and Daldrup-Link H E 2021 Glioblastoma multiforme (GBM): an overview of current therapies and mechanisms of resistance *Pharmacol. Res.* **171** 105780

[97] Urbańska K, Sokołowska J, Szmidt M and Sysa P 2014 Glioblastoma multiforme–an overview *Contemp. Oncol./Współcz. Onkol.* **18** 307–12

[98] Maier-Hauff K, Ulrich F, Nestler D, Niehoff H, Wust P, Thiesen B, Orawa H, Budach V and Jordan A 2011 Efficacy and safety of intratumoral thermotherapy using magnetic iron-oxide nanoparticles combined with external beam radiotherapy on patients with recurrent glioblastoma multiforme *J. Neuro-oncol.* **103** 317–24

[99] Dawson L A, Normolle D, Balter J M, McGinn C J, Lawrence T S and Ten Haken R K 2002 Analysis of radiation-induced liver disease using the Lyman NTCP model *Int. J. Radiat. Oncol. Biol. Phys.* **53** 810–21

[100] Jun B G, Kim Y D, Cheon G J, Kim E S, Jwa E, Kim S G, Kim Y S, Kim B S, Jeong S W and Jang J Y 2018 Clinical significance of radiation-induced liver disease after stereotactic body radiation therapy for hepatocellular carcinoma *Korean J. Int. Med.* **33** 1093

[101] Matsumine A, Takegami K, Asanuma K, Matsubara T, Nakamura T, Uchida A and Sudo A 2011 A novel hyperthermia treatment for bone metastases using magnetic materials *Int. J. Clin. Oncol.* **16** 101–8

[102] Beird H C, Bielack S S, Flanagan A M, Gill J, Heymann D, Janeway K A, Livingston J A, Roberts R D, Strauss S J and Gorlick R 2022 Osteosarcoma *Nat. Rev. Dis. Prim.* **8** 77

[103] Sadykova L R, Ntekim A I, Muyangwa-Semenova M, Rutland C S, Jeyapalan J N, Blatt N and Rizvanov A A 2020 Epidemiology and risk factors of osteosarcoma *Cancer Invest.* **38** 259–69

[104] Shirzadfar H and Khanahmadi M 2018 Current approaches and novel treatment methods for cancer and radiotherapy *Int. J. Biosens. Bioelectron.* **4** 224–9

[105] Liu T, Yang K and Liu Z 2020 Recent advances in functional nanomaterials for *x*-ray triggered cancer therapy *Prog. Nat. Sci.: Mater. Int.* **30** 567–76

[106] Clement S, Campbell J M, Deng W, Guller A, Nisar S, Liu G, Wilson B C and Goldys E M 2020 Mechanisms for tuning engineered nanomaterials to enhance radiation therapy of cancer *Adv. Sci.* **7** 2003584

[107] Kotb S, Detappe A, Lux F, Appaix F, Barbier E L, Tran V-L, Plissonneau M, Gehan H, Lefranc F and Rodriguez-Lafrasse C 2016 Gadolinium-based nanoparticles and radiation therapy for multiple brain melanoma metastases: proof of concept before phase I trial *Theranostics* **6** 418

[108] Verry C, Sancey L, Dufort S, Le Duc G, Mendoza C, Lux F, Grand S, Arnaud J, Quesada J L and Villa J 2019 Treatment of multiple brain metastases using gadolinium nanoparticles and radiotherapy: NANO-RAD, a phase I study protocol *BMJ Open* **9** e023591

[109] Wang J, Pan J, Tang Y, Chen J, Fei X, Xue W and Liu X 2023 Advances of hafnium based nanomaterials for cancer theranostics *Front. Chem.* **11** 1283924

[110] Skrodzki D, Molinaro M, Brown R, Moitra P and Pan D 2024 Synthesis and bioapplication of emerging nanomaterials of Hafnium *ACS Nano* **18** 1289–324

[111] Stergioula A, Pantelis E, Kontogeorgakos V, Lazaris A C and Agrogiannis G 2023 Understanding the role of radio-sensitizing nanoparticles in enhancing pathologic response in soft tissue sarcomas *Cancers* **15** 5572

[112] Wang J, Chen M, Chen C, Zheng B, Wang R, Guo Y, Wang Y, Jiang X and Long J 2024 Advancements in radiotherapy: the role of metal nanomaterials in enhancing therapeutic outcomes *J. Phys. Ther. Rehabil.* **1** 1003

[113] Hoffmann C *et al* 2021 Phase I dose-escalation study of NBTXR3 activated by intensity-modulated radiation therapy in elderly patients with locally advanced squamous cell carcinoma of the oral cavity or oropharynx *Eur. J. Cancer* **146** 135–44

[114] Maury P *et al* 2023 Clinical transfer of AGuIX®-based radiation treatments for locally advanced cervical cancer: MR quantification and *in vitro* insights in the NANOCOL clinical trial framework *Nanomed. Nanotechnol. Biol. Med.* **50** 102676

[115] Rarokar N, Yadav S, Saoji S, Bramhe P, Agade R, Gurav S, Khedekar P, Subramaniyan V, Wong L S and Kumarasamy V 2024 Magnetic nanosystem a tool for targeted delivery and diagnostic application: Current challenges and recent advancement *Int. J. Pharm.:* X **7** 100231

[116] Shava B, Ayodeji F D, Rahdar A, Iqbal H M and Bilal M 2022 Magnetic nanoparticles-based systems for multifaceted biomedical applications *J. Drug Deliv. Sci. Technol.* **74** 103616

[117] Babincova M and Babinec P 2009 Magnetic drug delivery and targeting: principles and applications *Biomed. Pap. Med. Fac. Univ. Palacky Olomouc Czech Repub.* **153** 243–50

[118] Bonnemain B 1998 Superparamagnetic agents in magnetic resonance imaging: physicochemical characteristics and clinical applications a review *J. Drug Target.* **6** 167–74

[119] Mornet S, Vasseur S, Grasset F and Duguet E 2004 Magnetic nanoparticle design for medical diagnosis and therapy *J. Mater. Chem.* **14** 2161–75

[120] Bauer J and Thorat N D 2022 Active magnetic nanoparticles, method of obtaining magnetic nanoparticles, medical and diagnostic use of magnetic nanoparticles und use as a carrier of biologically active agents and drugs, especially in tumors treatment, especially in cancers included breast cancer *European Patent* EP3960200A1

[121] lee K Y, Kim M S, Kim T H and Vu N P 2022 Metal oxide nanoparticle-based magnetic resonance imaging contrast agent with a central cavity *US Patent* US11324841B2

[122] Huang X and Bhana S 2018 Iron oxide-gold core–shell nanoparticles and uses thereof *US Patent* US9952209B2

[123] Ghosh S and Mitra S G 2021 Multimodal therapy for cancer cell destruction *US Patent* US11077191B2

[124] Mabray M C, Hetts S W, Lillaney P V, Losey A D, Jordan C D, Kondapavulur S and Cote A M 2018 Magnetic filtration devices and methods related thereto *US Patent* US10828414B2

[125] Zhenzhong Z, Luyang Z, Jinjin S, Wei L, Huifang Z *et al* 2018 Preparation method of mesoporous manganese dioxide nano drug-loading system with photodynamic therapy switching effect and molecular recognition effect *China Patent* CN107899013B

[126] Bae S and Chan J 2020 Giant self-heating alkali metal or alkaline earth metal-doped iron oxide nanoparticles in a biocompatible alternating magnetic field and method for producing the same *Japan Patent* JP2019536716A

[127] Xiaohui C 2019 A kind of novel pH Sensitive magnetic targeted nanometer medicine-carried system and its preparation method and application *China Patent* CN109953973A

[128] Kidd B L, Morris S C and Sabo M E 2019 Determination of structure and traversal of occlusions using magnetic particles *US Patent* US11918315B2
[129] Fei X, Xiuhong S, Ning G, Wei Q and Akira R 2019 Preparation method of iron oxide nanoparticles and application of iron oxide nanoparticles in tumor targeted diagnosis and treatment *China Patent* CN109125742B
[130] Jeonghoon, In-sook L and Young L 2023 Photothermal magnetic nanoparticle and preparing method thereof *Korea Patent* KR102527690B1
[131] Jie T, Jie H, Huihui, Jing Z, Zhenchao T and Yasuba 2022 Magnetic particle-based fieldfree line scanning imaging and field-free point positioning thermotherapy fusion device *China Patent* CN114521882B
[132] Quding, Yan C, Yuping L, Mengmeng H and Congyan L 2020 Traditional chinese medicine-magnetic nano-cluster chemical immunity drug delivery system and preparation method therefore *Patent* WO2020034696A1
[133] Aiguo W, Tianxiang C, Xuehua M, Ruifen Z, Zuber and Lingchao X 2020 Magnetic nano particle and preparation method and application thereof *China Patent* CN106913885B
[134] Seong-hoon K and Hye-min G 2019 Magnetic field driven therapy device and method *Korea Patent* KR102087825B1
[135] Copty A 2018 Localized hyperthermia/thermal ablation for cancer treatment *US Patent* US20180050218A1
[136] Aiguo W, Yuanyuan M, Tianxiang C and Fang Y 2019 Metal-doped ferrite nano material, preparation method of magnetic nano particles containing metal-doped ferrite nano material and application of magnetic nano particles *China Patent* CN109626439B
[137] Nan H, Haisong T and Yanlei L 2021 Nano diagnosis and treatment agent, preparation method and application *China Patent* CN112957467A
[138] Cheng K K, Kwok S K C, Ko C H, Tsai K and Ng C F 2019 Magnetic nanoparticles for disease diagnostics *US Patent* US10179179B2
[139] Dangpei L and Yanlei L 2019 Overstable monodispersed fluorescence magnetic diagnosis and treatment nano-probe and its preparation method and application *US Patent* CN109453395A
[140] Tishin A M, Pyatakov A P, Shtil A A, Gunko Y K, Zverev V I, Salakhova R T and Markova A A 2017 Method for treatment of malignant new-formations by magnetic hyperthermia and pharmaceutical compositions for application in indicated method *Russia Patent* RU2633918C2
[141] Khandhar A P, Krishnan K M, Ferguson R M and Kemp S 2017 Coated magnetic nanoparticles *US Patent* US9555136B2
[142] Ostrovska L 2021 Method for tumor detection and targeted hyperthermia *US Patent* US20210300754A1
[143] Peyman G A 2021 Cancer treatment and imaging methods using thermotherapy and drug delivery *US Patent* US20210220480A1
[144] Ruiz-Rincón S, González-Orive A, Grazú V, Fratila R M, de la Fuente J M and Cea P 2020 Altering model cell membranes by means of localized magnetic heating *Colloids Surf., B* **196** 111315
[145] Shah R R, Dombrowsky A R, Paulson A L, Johnson M P, Nikles D E and Brazel C S 2016 Determining iron oxide nanoparticle heating efficiency and elucidating local nanoparticle temperature for application in agarose gel-based tumor model *Mater. Sci. Eng.* C **68** 18–29

[146] Groth-Pedersen L and Jäättelä M 2013 Combating apoptosis and multidrug resistant cancers by targeting lysosomes *Cancer Lett.* **332** 265–74
[147] Sanchez C, El Hajj Diab D, Connord V, Clerc P, Meunier E, Pipy B, Payre B, Tan R P, Gougeon M and Carrey J 2014 Targeting a G-protein-coupled receptor overexpressed in endocrine tumors by magnetic nanoparticles to induce cell death *ACS Nano* **8** 1350–63
[148] Bunderson-Schelvan M, Holian A and Hamilton Jr R F 2017 Engineered nanomaterial-induced lysosomal membrane permeabilization and anti-cathepsin agents *J. Toxicol. Environ. Health, Part* B **20** 230–48
[149] Levada K, Pshenichnikov S, Omelyanchik A, Rodionova V, Nikitin A, Savchenko A, Schetinin I, Zhukov D, Abakumov M and Majouga A 2020 Progressive lysosomal membrane permeabilization induced by iron oxide nanoparticles drives hepatic cell autophagy and apoptosis *Nano Converg.* **7** 1–17
[150] Connord V, Clerc P, Hallali N, El Hajj Diab D, Fourmy D, Gigoux V and Carrey J 2015 Real-time analysis of magnetic hyperthermia experiments on living cells under a confocal microscope *Small* **11** 2437–45
[151] Clerc P, Jeanjean P, Hallali N, Gougeon M, Pipy B, Carrey J, Fourmy D and Gigoux V 2018 Targeted magnetic intra-lysosomal hyperthermia produces lysosomal reactive oxygen species and causes caspase-1 dependent cell death *J. Control. Release* **270** 120–34
[152] Appelqvist H, Johansson A-C, Linderoth E, Johansson U, Antonsson B, Steinfeld R, Kågedal K and Öllinger K 2012 Lysosome-mediated apoptosis is associated with cathepsin D-specific processing of bid at Phe24, Trp48, and Phe183 *Ann. Clin. Lab. Sci.* **42** 231–42
[153] Chidambaranathan-Reghupaty S, Fisher P B and Sarkar D 2021 Hepatocellular carcinoma (HCC): epidemiology, etiology and molecular classification *Adv. Cancer Res.* **149** 1–61
[154] Rumgay H, Ferlay J, de Martel C, Georges D, Ibrahim A S, Zheng R, Wei W, Lemmens V E and Soerjomataram I 2022 Global, regional and national burden of primary liver cancer by subtype *Eur. J. Cancer* **161** 108–18
[155] Zeng L, Gowda B J, Ahmed M G, Abourehab M A, Chen Z-S, Zhang C, Li J and Kesharwani P 2023 Advancements in nanoparticle-based treatment approaches for skin cancer therapy *Mol. Cancer* **22** 10
[156] Ahmed B, Qadir M I and Ghafoor S 2020 Malignant melanoma: skin cancer– diagnosis, prevention, and treatment *Crit. Rev. Eukaryot. Gene Expr.* **30** 291–97
[157] Kallini J R, Hamed N and Khachemoune A 2015 Squamous cell carcinoma of the skin: epidemiology, classification, management, and novel trends *Int. J. Dermatol.* **54** 130–40
[158] Xu Y G, Aylward J L, Swanson A M, Spiegelman V S, Vanness E R, Teng J M, Snow S N and Wood G S 2020 Nonmelanoma skin cancers: basal cell and squamous cell carcinomas *Abeloff's Clinical Oncology* (Amsterdam: Elsevier) pp 1052–73.e8
[159] Bakos R M, Blumetti T P, Roldán-Marín R and Salerni G 2018 Noninvasive imaging tools in the diagnosis and treatment of skin cancers *Am. J. Clin. Dermatol.* **19** 3–14
[160] Jain S and Pise N 2015 Computer aided melanoma skin cancer detection using image processing *Procedia Comp. Sci.* **48** 735–40
[161] Mahmoud N M and Soliman A M 2024 Early automated detection system for skin cancer diagnosis using artificial intelligent techniques *Sci. Rep.* **14** 9749
[162] Fang S and Salven P 2011 Stem cells in tumor angiogenesis *J. Mol. Cell. Cardiol.* **50** 290–5
[163] Zhao L, Li Q, Zhou T, Liu X, Guo J, Fang Q, Cao X, Geng Q, Yu Y and Zhang S 2024 Role of N6-methyladenosine in tumor neovascularization *Cell Death Dis.* **15** 563

[164] Lv S, Liu Y, Xie C, Xue C, Du S and Yao J 2023 Emerging role of interactions between tumor angiogenesis and cancer stem cells *J. Control. Release* **360** 468–81
[165] Motomura K, Izumi T, Tateishi S, Tamaki Y, Ito Y, Horinouchi T and Nakanishi K 2016 Superparamagnetic iron oxide-enhanced MRI at 3 T for accurate axillary staging in breast cancer *J. Br. Surg.* **103** 60–9

IOP Publishing

Magnetic Nanomaterials
Innovation for cancer theranostics

Sudip Mukherjee, Vijay Sagar Madamsetty, Lipi Pradhan, Anjali Upadhyay and Devyani Yenurkar

Chapter 6

Magnetic nanoparticles: biodistribution, excretion, toxicity, and overall conclusions

Magnetic nanoparticles (MNPs) have gained immense attention due to their multifunctional biomedical applications, such as MRI imaging, photothermal therapy, drug delivery, cancer immunotherapy, anticancer therapy, and magnetic hyperthermia (MHT). It is necessary to highlight the biodistribution and organ-specific accumulation of MNPs, as their long-term toxicity is an important factor in their use, immunogenicity, and excretion route. This chapter highlights these topics and offers overall conclusions.

MNPs have attracted immense attention due to their multifunctional biomedical applications, such as MRI imaging, photothermal therapy, drug delivery, cancer immunotherapy, anticancer therapy, MHT, etc (figure 6.1).

Evaluation of the *in vivo* pharmacokinetics of injected MNPs, along with their extent of biodistribution to various organs, rate of biodegradation and excretion, short- and long-term toxicity, and immunogenicity, is essential for the effective clinical translation of these nanoformulations. In this chapter, we discuss various physiological and biological properties of MNPs and establish the importance of these properties.

6.1 Biodistribution and excretion of MNPs

It is essential to analyze the biodistribution of injected nanoparticles (NPs) aimed at treating certain diseases. In general, the size, shape, surface charge, nature of the coating, tendency to aggregate, and interaction with immune cells play crucial roles in dictating the biodistribution of these NPs to target specific sites. More often, inefficiency in targeting has significantly hindered NPs from reaching the target disease site, reducing the potential for successful treatment. The biodistribution of MNPs depends on different physicochemical properties, including hydrodynamic size, nature of aggregation, shape, surface charge, surface coating, protein corona

doi:10.1088/978-0-7503-6335-8ch6 © IOP Publishing Ltd 2025. All rights, including for text and data mining (TDM), artificial intelligence (AI) training, and similar technologies, are reserved.

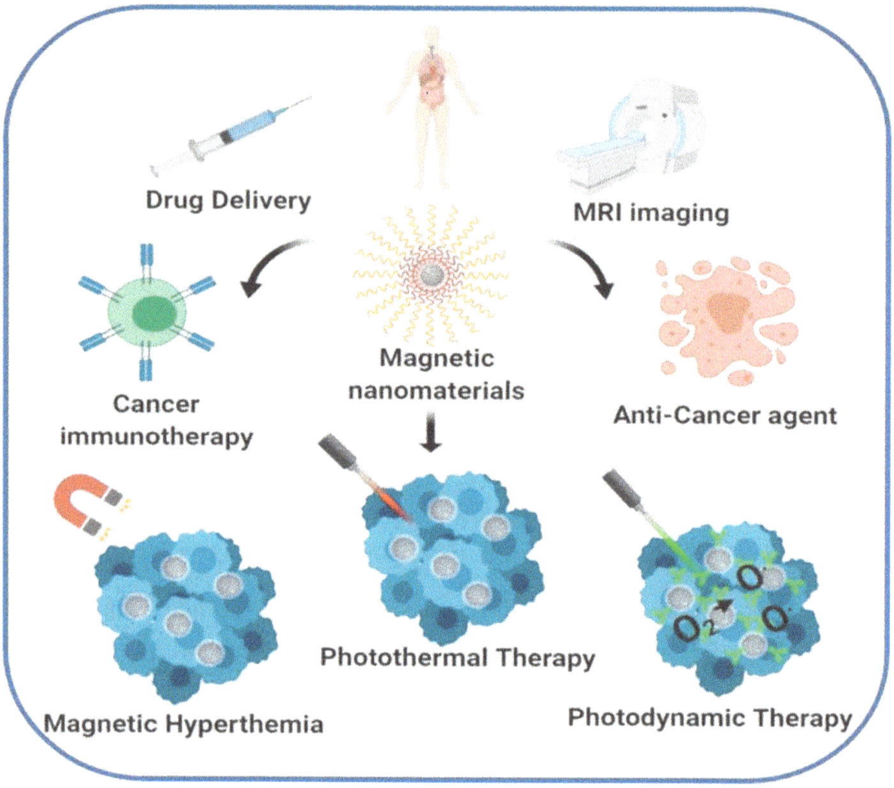

Figure 6.1. Multifunctional biomedical applications of MNPs. Adapted from [1]. CC BY 4.0.

formation, and interaction of MNPs with the reticuloendothelial system (RES), also known as the mononuclear phagocytic system (MPS) [2].

Liver: specific macrophages named Kupffer cells make up a significant part of the liver and are the largest macrophage cell population in human tissues (figure 6.2) [3]. Kupffer cells are crucial, playing a vital role in the human body's immune response by proficiently engulfing pathogens and other particles larger than 100 nm in the blood circulation [4]. The conjugation of targeting ligands such as linoleic acid and polyethylene glycol (PEG) can enhance the uptake of Kupffer cells through cell-specific targeting agents or antifouling molecules [5].

Tate *et al* analyzed the biodistribution of hydroxyl-ethyl starch-coated magnetite NPs with sizes of 20 and 110 nm in a mouse model for an injected dose of 80 mg Fe/kg mouse [6]. The biodistribution results demonstrated a higher accumulation of MNPs in the liver and spleen in various time-dependent manners (4, 24, and 72 h); for 110 nm MNPs, approximately 1.6 mg Fe/g tissue was detected. The iron level stayed elevated until day 14, gradually decreased over time, and was similar to the control level by day 580. However, other important organs, including the brain, lungs, and heart, did not show significant accumulation of MNPs. Moreover, it was observed that at a size of

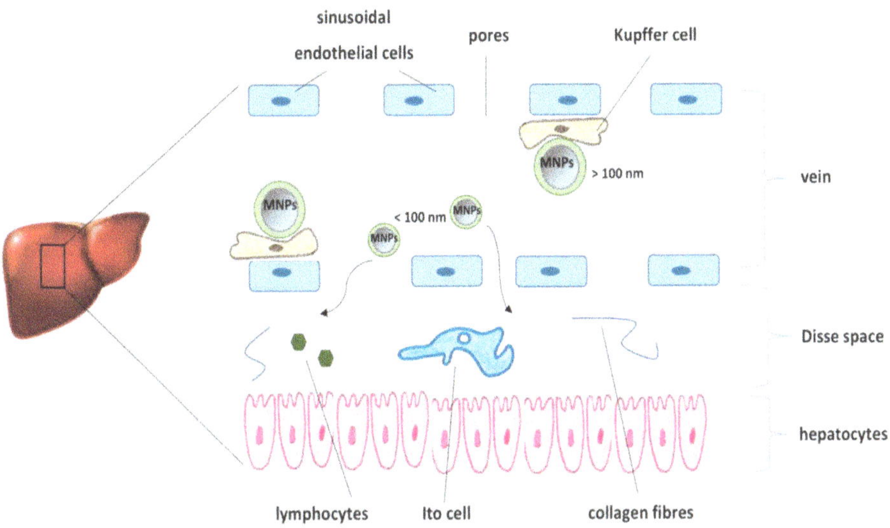

Figure 6.2. In the liver, Kupffer cells can quickly take up large NPs (>100 nm), whereas smaller NPs (<100 nm) are captured in the Disse space, from where, if suitably functionalized, they can also accumulate in hepatocytes. Reproduced with permission from [2]. © 2023, The Author(s), CC BY-NC 3.0. Dove Medical Press Limited reprinted by permission of Informa UK Limited, trading as Taylor & Francis Ltd, https://www.tandfonline.com.

110 nm, MNPs had a higher accumulation in the liver compared to the smaller MNPs (20 nm) at all time points.

Shanehsazzadeh *et al* examined the organ distribution of MRI-active ultrasmall iron oxide NPs labeled with the radioisotope technetium-99m in a model of BALB/c mice [7]. NPs with a size of 41 nm were injected intravenously, and a surprising 75% of the iron oxide NPs gathered in the liver and spleen 15 min after injection. However, around 24% of the injected dose remained in the liver 48 h post-injection, and only 3% of the distribution occurred in the spleen. In summary, these studies demonstrate that the liver is the primary filtration point where MNPs accumulate. Because of the high accumulation in the liver, iron oxide NPs have been effectively utilized as MRI T2 contrast agents for liver cancer diagnosis. In general, this is helpful in the sensing of liver tumors, as MNPs are captured by Kupffer cells in healthy parts of the liver, producing dark contrast in T2-weighted MRI. On the other hand, cancer cells not containing Kupffer cells appear as bright regions.

6.2 Conclusions

Research and development of MNPs for biological applications has significantly increased in recent years. Widespread research into the possible applications of these NPs has been spurred by the ability to precisely manipulate their size, shape, and surface properties. Among the many benefits of MNPs are their potential for use in therapies such as hyperthermia and their ability to be precisely targeted to particular bodily areas through an alternating magnetic field. MNPs permit significant replacement levels due to their high surface-area-to-volume ratio, which makes them ideal for medication delivery. Additionally, their addition to composites such as liposomes or magnetic hydrogels creates new classes of multipurpose hybrid nanostructures that are more biocompatible and have a wider range of potential medical uses. In addition to these uses, they have also been thought to be beneficial in tissue engineering and regenerative medicine. Future studies and developments in these areas should open the door to more individualized and efficient biomedical treatments employing MNPs. Beyond their fundamental magnetic characteristics, smart MNPs (SMNPs) have further uses. These structures can be used for regulated and directed targeted drug delivery (TDD), MHT, magnetic resonance imaging (MRI), and magnetofection (MF) applications, since they can made to react to particular stimuli or situations. Furthermore, inside the body, these MNPs can be remotely activated and manipulated by external stimuli such as magnetic fields [8]. Because of their low toxicological profile and promising biocompatibility in oncology, iron-oxide-based MNPs such as Fe_3O_4 (magnetite) and γ-Fe_2O_3 (maghemite) are being investigated extensively. They can be used as MRI contrast agents, among other applications. To ensure MNPs are readily adopted and have a significant near-term impact on clinical use and theranostics, current research is concentrating on enhancing the surface properties and biocompatible coatings of MNPs to decrease their toxicity and improve their drug-holding capacity, specificity, and affinity toward target tumor cells. Although several gold-coated or iron-based MNPs have promising multifunctional medical spectra (as optical imaging agents in PTT and MRI) for cancer therapy, they also offer theranostic advantages [9].

Several issues constrain the industry's production of MNPs. These restrictions result from the synthesis process's intricacy, the requirement for consistency and scalability, and concerns about costs, security, and the environment. Toxicology is the central area of concern when considering MNPs for future medical applications because scant research has been conducted. Toxicity studies typically describe the negative impacts of testing on animals or the surrounding ecosystem through the lens of physical, chemical, and biological agents. These toxic particles may also cause reduced therapeutic efficacy and MNP migration and deposition in organs, triggering immunological or inflammatory reactions. These MNPs can infiltrate cells, where their toxicity may impact nuclear processes, result in leakage from the membrane, or cause obstruction, which may negatively affect cell survival, proliferation, or metabolic activity. Damage to the cytoskeleton during incubation with anionic NPs hindered neurite development and significantly reduced the length of the neurites and the number of neurite forms per cell [10].

MNPs are attracting much attention for use in biological medicine, including drug administration, imaging, and diagnostics, because of their tiny size, surface characteristics, and potential for functionalization. However, their use may cause issues related to immunogenicity. When foreign particles, including NPs with magnetic properties, are not adequately functionalized, the human body's immune system cells, including macrophages, can identify and absorb them. As a result, NPs may be quickly removed from the circulatory system and unable to reach their intended target. The way that MNPs communicate with the body's immune system is significantly influenced by their surface characteristics, including charge, hydrophobicity, and the material used for the coating. Immunogenicity may result if improper surface coatings are recognized by complement proteins or immune system cells. When compared to ionic NPs, it was discovered that citrate-coated NPs significantly raised the mitotic index of peritoneal macrophages, triggering an immunological response. By increasing the number of lymphocytes in the intra-peritoneal cell population, both types of NPs caused an inflammatory reaction. Furthermore, the nuclei of neutrophils and lymphocytes were significantly harmed by increased amounts of these ionic or citrate-coated NPs, suggesting that these two types of NPs are hazardous after intraperitoneal delivery, which may indicate a form of intravenous administration [11].

MNPs have enormous potential for use in biological domains such as imaging, targeted administration of drugs, and MHT. However, their efficacy and clinical translation are significantly impacted by the difficulties presented by their engagement with biological systems. The process by which plasma proteins (opsonins) attach to the surface of NPs, referred to as NP opsonization, continues to be the principal barrier among these difficulties. One effective tactic for combating opsonization involves surface functionalization [12]. Applying a polyethylene glycol (PEG) coating to MNPs is one of the most investigated techniques. The PEG surrounds the NPs with a steric and hydrophilic barrier that inhibits immunological identification and protein adhesion. For example, PEGylated MNPs used in drug delivery systems show decreased macrophage absorption *in vivo* and longer blood circulation durations [13]. Because of their capacity to withstand nonspecific adhesion to proteins while preserving biocompatibility, zwitterionic polymers with both positive and negative charges have attracted interest in addition to PEG. According to studies, zwitterion-coated MNPs have improved stealth qualities, guaranteeing more effective delivery of therapeutic payloads [14].

Despite these developments, improving surface coatings to balance usefulness, biocompatibility, and the maintenance of magnetic characteristics still presents difficulties. Additionally, surface changes have to maintain the structural integrity of the NPs while withstanding physiological conditions, including enzyme activity and mechanical stress. While achieving site-specific targeting is essential, it presents a challenge: incorporating targeting ligands may unintentionally enhance opsonization, since proteins may bind to these ligands. These problems can be solved creatively by creating biomimetic or stimuli-responsive coatings. For instance, coating MNPs with cell membrane fragments has demonstrated the potential to enhance targeting effectiveness and avoid immune system recognition [15, 16]. Although NP opsonization by surface engineering has advanced significantly, further study is required to improve these approaches. Developing multifunctional coatings that minimize immune recognition, ensure stability, and maintain functionality under diverse physiological conditions is essential.

The clinical utility of MNPs is often impeded by rapid clearance through the MPS. The MPS, mostly made up of macrophages found in the lymph nodes, liver, and spleen, is essential for identifying and removing foreign particles from the bloodstream [17]. This clearing process primarily marks MNPs for phagocytosis by triggering opsonization on their surface. As a result, the therapeutic efficacy of

MNPs is severely compromised due to reduced bioavailability and altered biodistribution. One major obstacle to advancing MNP-based biological applications is overcoming MPS-mediated clearance [18]. By changing their biodistribution, lowering their therapeutic payload, and hindering their capacity to target tumors efficiently, the MPS substantially negatively influences the effectiveness of MNPs in cancer treatment [19]. For example, proteins such as complement and immunoglobulins quickly opsonize iron oxide NPs utilized in breast cancer drug delivery, indicating their removal by spleen macrophages and liver Kupffer cells. The efficacy of treatments like chemotherapy or hyperthermia is lowered because of this quick clearance, which reduces the concentration of MNPs that may accumulate at the tumor site [20]. MNPs utilized in MHT are used to produce localized heat that destroys cancer cells. However, research has revealed that a significant percentage of these MNPs end up in the liver and spleen rather than the tumor, resulting in inadequate therapeutic results [21]. Furthermore, enhanced opsonin binding to ligands might compromise TDD based on ligand-functionalized MNPs, such as folic-acid-conjugated NPs for ovarian cancer, by improving macrophage detection and clearance. Even when drug-loaded MNPs reach their target, the immune activation caused by MPS interactions can trigger inflammation, further complicating treatment and potentially affecting the tumor microenvironment [22]. To overcome these obstacles and enhance the therapeutic effectiveness of MNPs in cancer treatment, novel approaches such as PEGylation or biomimetic coatings are required.

However, the nonspecific distribution of MNPs can significantly compromise therapeutic outcomes and pose potential risks. For instance, MNPs may accumulate in healthy tissues such as the liver, spleen, or lungs due to the natural clearance mechanisms of the RES. These organs may experience toxicity or inflammation due to this nonspecific absorption [23]. Additionally, uneven distribution within the tumor can result in suboptimal hyperthermia during MHT therapy, where localized heating is used to destroy cancer cells. For example, MNPs trapped in peripheral regions of the tumor might leave the tumor core untreated, enabling cancer cells to survive and proliferate. Moreover, in drug delivery applications, nonspecific distribution reduces the concentration of therapeutic agents reaching the tumor, lowering treatment efficacy. To overcome these challenges, researchers are exploring surface modification of MNPs with biocompatible coatings or conjugation with targeting ligands like antibodies or peptides to improve their specificity and minimize off-target effects.

Cellular internalization plays a crucial role in the efficacy of MNPs in cancer therapy, particularly in TDD and MHT. Once administered, MNPs must successfully penetrate cancer cells to deliver therapeutic agents or induce localized heat under an external magnetic field [24]. The internalization process, influenced by particle size, surface charge, coating materials, and functionalization with targeting ligands, directly determines MNPs^ therapeutic outcomes [25]. For instance, MNPs functionalized with folic acid target folate receptors overexpressed on cancer cells, enhancing their uptake via receptor-mediated endocytosis. The efficiency of this internalization affects both drug delivery and hyperthermia effectiveness. In drug delivery, poorly internalized NPs may release drugs prematurely in the extracellular environment, reducing specificity and causing toxicity to healthy tissues. In MHT, MNPs that fail to internalize adequately may not achieve sufficient intracellular heating to induce cancer cell apoptosis. Studies have demonstrated that MNPs with optimal sizes and hydrophilic coatings improve cellular uptake while minimizing aggregation in the bloodstream. Additionally, modifying MNP surfaces with peptides or antibodies enhances their selectivity, ensuring they concentrate in cancer cells rather than being cleared by the immune system [26]. Thus, understanding and optimizing cellular internalization mechanisms are pivotal for maximizing the therapeutic potential of MNPs in cancer therapy. These advancements could lead to more efficient, targeted treatments with reduced side effects.

However, once these NPs are internalized by cells through endocytosis, they are typically trapped within endosomes. Without an escape, the therapeutic payload remains confined in these endosomal vesicles and may eventually be degraded in lysosomes, reducing the therapy's efficacy [27]. For example, MNPs functionalized with pH-responsive polymers, such as polyethylenimine (PEI), can exploit the endosomes' acidic environment to destabilize the endosomal membrane, releasing the payload into the cytoplasm. This endosomal escape mechanism ensures that therapeutic agents reach their intracellular targets effectively. These agents include small interfering RNA (siRNA) that targets oncogenic pathways and chemotherapeutic drugs like doxorubicin. Additionally, external magnetic fields can enhance the targeting and penetration capabilities of MNPs, but their success still hinges on efficient endosomal escape to overcome intracellular barriers. Researchers can significantly enhance therapeutic outcomes in cancer treatments by improving the design of MNPs to promote endosomal escape, for example, by incorporating fusogenic peptides or membrane-disrupting agents.

Drug efflux pumps, such as P-glycoprotein (P-gp) and multidrug-resistance-associated proteins (MRPs), pose a significant challenge in cancer therapy by actively expelling therapeutic agents from cancer cells, reducing drug efficacy [28]. These efflux pumps can diminish the therapeutic potential of MNPs employed as drug delivery systems. For example, MNPs loaded with chemotherapeutic drugs such as doxorubicin are designed to deliver drugs directly to tumor cells under an external magnetic field. However, even after successful delivery, the drugs released by the NPs can be ejected by efflux pumps, resulting in subtherapeutic intracellular drug concentrations. This mechanism often leads to multidrug resistance (MDR), a common obstacle in cancer treatment. To counteract this, researchers are developing MNPs functionalized with efflux pump inhibitors, such as verapamil or tariquidar, to block pump activity. By codelivering these inhibitors alongside the chemotherapeutic agents, MNPs can enhance drug retention and potency within cancer cells, improving treatment outcomes [29]. With continued advancements in materials science and nanotechnology, the full potential of MNPs in biomedical applications can be realized, paving the way for more effective diagnostics and therapies.

Multidisciplinary studies in nanomedicine have witnessed significant advancements in developing MNPs and optimizing their surface properties, making remarkable progress in cancer theranostics. However, FDA authorization for the therapeutic application of MNPs continues to be limited, and the progression from laboratory testing to clinical trials is undoubtedly slow. Future studies could focus on improving the formulation of MNPs to boost their targeting abilities and extend their use in various types of cancer. Such advances could increase the specificity of MNPs for tumor sites, facilitating the efficient delivery of therapeutic agents while reducing undesirable side effects. Additionally, combining MNPs with cutting-edge imaging techniques could significantly increase the effectiveness of treatment by offering real-time monitoring through modern imaging methods, enabling personalized cancer therapies. The personalization of treatment for cancer may also be entirely transformed by combining MNPs with advanced technologies like machine learning (ML) and artificial intelligence (AI). To make treatments more effective and patient-specific, AI and ML algorithms can analyze large databases to find trends, predict treatment outcomes, and optimize strategies for treatment. Another exciting avenue is building multimodal platforms that integrate MNPs with different imaging methods, such as optical, ultrasound, and nuclear imaging. These platforms would improve our understanding of tumor progression and treatment effectiveness by offering a thorough approach to therapeutic and diagnostic monitoring. The future of MNPs in cancer theranostics additionally includes strengthening their capacity for specific drug delivery, enhancing their effectiveness in overcoming drug resistance, and combining multifaceted strategies for treatment. Moving MNPs to the clinical testing phase should be the primary objective of future research to facilitate their incorporation into commercial applications for the benefit of society.

Future research should also focus on understanding the long-term effects of MNPs on the human body after they have served their functional purpose, which is an essential but frequently disregarded factor. MNPs can gradually build up in body tissues because they are not biodegradable. This presents serious questions about their interactions with biological systems, post-functional behavior, final destiny, and excretion pathways. To thoroughly examine these factors, extensive long-term research is necessary. Addressing these issues will improve their acceptability and dependability in the medical and business sectors and open the door for their successful use in cancer treatment. MNPs can also be coated using bioinspired and biomimetic compounds resembling biological interfaces, shielding them from immune recognition, prolonging their bloodstream circulation, and improving their delivery to target sites. The efficiency and adaptability of MNPs in biomedical applications can be significantly increased using sophisticated fabrication techniques like layer-by-layer assembly, microfluidic-assisted synthesis, and 3D bioprinting. These techniques can precisely control the shape, size, and surface chemistry of MNPs, enhancing their therapeutic efficacy and scalability in clinical settings. MNPs can also be incorporated into hydrogels or 3D-printed scaffolds, making the release of local and controllable therapeutic agents easier.

A multimodal approach can also be designed by combining immunotherapy, chemotherapy, and hyperthermia into a single MNP system for synergistic therapeutic effects. Researchers can also design patient-specific approaches to increase efficacy by customizing MNP formulations to each patient's unique genetic profile and tumor characteristics. Efforts are being made to create biodegradable MNPs that minimize harmful byproducts during their breakdown or clearance while reducing long-term accumulation in the body to address safety concerns. Researchers and engineers are pushing the limits of MNP-based cancer theranostics by continually designing new ideas and methods, opening the way to more individualized and efficient treatments for cancer.

References

[1] Mukherjee S, Liang L and Veiseh O 2020 Recent advancements of magnetic nanomaterials in cancer therapy *Pharmaceutics* **12** 147

[2] Nowak-Jary J and Machnicka B 2023 *In vivo* biodistribution and clearance of magnetic iron oxide nanoparticles for medical applications *Int. J. Nanomed.* **18** 4067–100

[3] Dixon L J, Barnes M, Tang H, Pritchard M T and Nagy L E 2013 Kupffer cells in the liver *Compr. Physiol.* **3** 785

[4] Gu L, Fang R H, Sailor M J and Park J-H 2012 *In vivo* clearance and toxicity of monodisperse iron oxide nanocrystals *ACS Nano* **6** 4947–54

[5] Lee C-M, Jeong H-J, Kim S-L, Kim E-M, Kim D W, Lim S T, Jang K Y, Jeong Y Y, Nah J-W and Sohn M-H 2009 SPION-loaded chitosan–linoleic acid nanoparticles to target hepatocytes *Int. J. Pharm.* **371** 163–9

[6] Tate J A, Petryk A A, Giustini A J and Hoopes P J 2011 *In vivo* biodistribution of iron oxide nanoparticles: an overview *Energy-based Treat. Tissue Assess. VI* **7901** 384–92

[7] Shanehsazzadeh S, Oghabian M A, Daha F J, Amanlou M and Allen B J 2013 Biodistribution of ultra small superparamagnetic iron oxide nanoparticles in BALB mice *J. Radioanal. Nucl. Chem.* **295** 1517–23

[8] Stiufiuc G F and Stiufiuc R I 2024 Magnetic nanoparticles: synthesis, characterization, and their use in biomedical field *Appl. Sci.* **14** 1623

[9] Sharma K and Chauhan C 2023 Role of magnetic nanoparticle (MNPs) in cancer treatment: a review *Mater. Today Proc.* **81** 919–25

[10] Chen Q, Liu L, Lu Y, Chen X, Zhang Y, Zhou W, Guo Q, Li C, Zhang Y and Zhang Y 2019 Tumor microenvironment-triggered aggregated magnetic nanoparticles for reinforced image-guided immunogenic chemotherapy *Adv. Sci.* **6** 1802134

[11] Reddy L H, Arias J L, Nicolas J and Couvreur P 2012 Magnetic nanoparticles: design and characterization, toxicity and biocompatibility, pharmaceutical and biomedical applications *Chem. Rev.* **112** 5818–78

[12] Shakeri-Zadeh A and Bulte J W 2024 Imaging-guided precision hyperthermia with magnetic nanoparticles *Nat. Rev. Bioeng.* **3** 245–60

[13] Wen H, Huo G, Qin C, Wu H, Wang D, Dan M, Geng X and Liu S 2023 Safety evaluation of PEGylated MNPs and p-PEGylated MNPs in SD rats *Sci. Rep.* **13** 21501

[14] Moayedi S, Xia W, Lundergan L, Yuan H and Xu J 2024 Zwitterionic polymers for biomedical applications: antimicrobial and antifouling strategies toward implantable medical devices and drug delivery *Langmuir* **40** 23125–45

[15] Liu L, Bai X, Martikainen M-V, Kårlund A, Roponen M, Xu W, Hu G, Tasciotti E and Lehto V-P 2021 Cell membrane coating integrity affects the internalization mechanism of biomimetic nanoparticles *Nat. Commun.* **12** 5726

[16] Oroojalian F, Beygi M, Baradaran B, Mokhtarzadeh A and Shahbazi M A 2021 Immune cell membrane-coated biomimetic nanoparticles for targeted cancer therapy *Small* **17** 2006484

[17] Zelepukin I V, Shevchenko K G and Deyev S M 2024 Rediscovery of mononuclear phagocyte system blockade for nanoparticle drug delivery *Nat. Commun.* **15** 4366
[18] Mills J A, Liu F, Jarrett T R, Fletcher N L and Thurecht K J 2022 Nanoparticle based medicines: approaches for evading and manipulating the mononuclear phagocyte system and potential for clinical translation *Biomater. Sci.* **10** 3029–53
[19] Dai X, Dai Y, Zheng Y and Lv Y 2024 Magnetic nanoparticles and possible synergies with cold atmospheric plasma for cancer treatment *RSC Adv.* **14** 29039–51
[20] Park S-J, Han S R, Kang Y H, Lee E-J, Kim E-G, Hong H, Jeong J-C, Lee M-S, Lee S-H and Song D-Y 2022 *In vivo* preclinical tumor-specific imaging of superparamagnetic iron oxide nanoparticles using magnetic particle imaging for cancer diagnosis *Int. J. Nanomed.* **17** 3711
[21] Cheng H W, Tsao H Y, Chiang C S and Chen S Y 2021 Advances in magnetic nanoparticle-mediated cancer immune-theranostics *Adv. Healthc. Mater.* **10** 2001451
[22] Patra A, Satpathy S, Naik P K, Kazi M and Hussain M D 2022 Folate receptor-targeted PLGA-PEG nanoparticles for enhancing the activity of genistein in ovarian cancer *Artif. Cells, Nanomed. Biotechnol.* **50** 228–39
[23] Li X, Li W, Wang M and Liao Z 2021 Magnetic nanoparticles for cancer theranostics: advances and prospects *J. Control. Release* **335** 437–48
[24] Sun W, Chai X, Zhang Y, Yu T, Wang Y, Zhao W, Liu Y, Yin D and Zhang C 2024 Combination using magnetic iron oxide nanoparticles and magnetic field for cancer therapy *Chem. Rec.* **24** e202400179
[25] Martín M J, Gentili C and Lassalle V 2020 *In vitro* biological tests as the first tools to validate magnetic nanotheranostics for colorectal cancer models *ChemMedChem* **15** 1003–17
[26] Setia A, Mehata A K, Malik A K, Viswanadh M K and Muthu M S 2023 Theranostic magnetic nanoparticles: synthesis, properties, toxicity, and emerging trends for biomedical applications *J. Drug Deliv. Sci. Technol.* **81** 104295
[27] Shirsat S D, Londhe P V, Gaikwad A P, Rizwan M, Laha S S, Khot V M, Achal V, Tabish T A and Thorat N D 2024 Endosomal escape in magnetic nanostructures: recent advances and future perspectives *Mater. Today Adv.* **22** 100484
[28] Yao Y, Zhou Y, Liu L, Xu Y, Chen Q, Wang Y, Wu S, Deng Y, Zhang J and Shao A 2020 Nanoparticle-based drug delivery in cancer therapy and its role in overcoming drug resistance *Front. Mol. Biosci.* **7** 193
[29] Gao L, Meng F, Yang Z, Lafuente-Merchan M, Fernández L M, Cao Y, Kusamori K, Nishikawa M, Itakura S and Chen J 2024 Nano-drug delivery system for the treatment of multidrug-resistant breast cancer: current status and future perspectives *Biomed. Pharmacother.* **179** 117327

www.ingramcontent.com/pod-product-compliance
Ingram Content Group UK Ltd.
Pitfield, Milton Keynes, MK11 3LW, UK
UKHW051852100926
8556IPUK00005B/590